American Academy of Orthopaedic Surgeons
6300 North River Road
Rosemont, Illinois 60018
1-800-626-6726

D1672100

The Female Athlete

EDITED BY
CAROL C. TEITZ, MD

Associate Professor, Orthopaedic Surgery
University of Washington
Seattle, Washington

CONTRIBUTORS
Elizabeth K. Arendt, MD
Carol Frey, MD
Serena S. Hu, MD
Suzanne M. Tanner, MD
Carol C. Teitz, MD

SERIES EDITOR
Glenn B. Pfeffer, MD

THE FEMALE ATHLETE
American Academy of
Orthopaedic Surgeons

The American Academy of Orthopaedic Surgeons Monograph Series is dedicated to Wendy O. Schmidt, American Academy of Orthopaedic Surgeons senior medical editor, 1987-1991.

The material presented in *The Female Athlete* has been made available by the American Academy of Orthopaedic Surgeons for educational purposes only. This material is not intended to present the only, or necessarily best, methods or procedures for the medical situations discussed, but rather is intended to represent an approach, view, statement, or opinion of the author(s) or producer(s), which may be helpful to others who face similar situations.

Some drugs and medical devices demonstrated in Academy courses or described in Academy print or electronic publications have Food and Drug Administration (FDA) clearance for use for specific purposes or for use only in restricted settings. The FDA has stated that it is the responsibility of the physician to determine the FDA status of each drug or device he or she wishes to use in clinical practice, and to use the products with appropriate patient consent and in compliance with applicable law.

At the time of this writing, bone screws placed posteriorly into vertebral elements have not been cleared for use in this specific manner by the Food and Drug Administration (FDA). These are Class III devices. This category includes screws placed transfacetally, within pedicles, or in articular, lateral masses. Some bone screws for use within the sacrum have been approved as Class II devices. Some companies have received Class II clearance for use of screws in lumbar pedicles specifically to supplement fusions in the treatment of grade III and IV spondylolisthesis with the proviso that these devices are removed after the arthrodesis has healed. Anterior vertebral body screws (cervical, thoracic, and lumbar) are Class II devices and can be used as labeled in vertebral bodies. Many of the posterior screw-based devices have been shown in laboratory and clinical testing to be useful and may be used in an off-label manner if the physician feels this is appropriate and important for the treatment of the patient. As with all surgeries, informed consent should explain the procedure and why a particular technique has been chosen, as well as its risks and benefits. The question of whether informed consent regarding pedicle screws must include a discussion of the device's FDA clearance status is currently being litigated in several jurisdictions. In cases that have been included in the multidistrict litigation in the Eastern District of Pennsylvania, this additional requirement has not been imposed.

Furthermore, any statements about commercial products are solely the opinion(s) of the author(s) and do not represent an Academy endorsement or evaluation of these products. These statements may not be used in advertising or for any commercial purpose.

The material contained in this volume was submitted as previously unpublished material, except in the instances in which credit has been given to the source from which some of the illustrative material was derived.

First Edition
Copyright © 1997 by the American Academy of Orthopaedic Surgeons

The Female Athlete
edited by Carol C. Teitz, MD

ISBN 0-89203-152-2

CONTENTS

CONTRIBUTORS

Elizabeth K. Arendt, MD
Associate Professor
Department of Orthopaedic Surgery
University of Minnesota
Minneapolis, Minnesota

Carol Frey, MD
Associate Clinical Professor
  of Orthopaedic Surgery
University of Southern California
Director, Orthopaedic Foot and Ankle Center
Orthopaedic Hospital Campus
Los Angeles, California

Serena S. Hu, MD
Assistant Professor
Department of Orthopaedic Surgery
University of California, San Francisco
San Francisco, California

Suzanne M. Tanner, MD
Assistant Professor
Departments of Orthopaedics and Pediatrics
University of Colorado
  Health Sciences Center
Denver, Colorado

Carol C. Teitz, MD
Associate Professor
Department of Orthopaedic Surgery
University of Washington
Seattle, Washington

PREFACE

Women were first permitted to participate in the Olympic games in 1900 in tennis and golf. However, it wasn't until 1984 that women were allowed to run the marathon. Title IX was signed into law in 1975 requiring accommodation of both men's and women's interests and abilities, athletic benefits and opportunities, and financial assistance.[1] Before the passage of Title IX, only 7% of interscholastic athletes were women. Since then, the numbers of girls and women participating in recreational, interscholastic, intercollegiate, and Olympic sports have skyrocketed.

This increasing participation has brought to the forefront concerns about the effects of intense exercise on the female athlete. These concerns include heat tolerance, effects on fertility and the fetus, and musculoskeletal problems. Properly training and equipping the female athlete is also an issue. Progress has been made in some areas. For example, it now is known that thermal stress is not gender dependent and the key to withstanding it is conditioning. In other areas, though, there still is much research to do. Delayed menarche and menstrual abnormalities associated with vigorous exercise were recognized in the early 1970s. However, these findings did not generate widespread concern until 1984 when Cann and associates[2] first described osteoporosis in young amenorrheic athletes. In 1991, the American College of Sports Medicine convened a task force on women's issues in sports medicine, and the term "the female athlete triad" was coined to describe the complex interplay of disordered eating, menstrual irregularity, and osteoporosis seen in the female athlete.[3] It is not yet known whether the loss in bone mineral density at a young age will lead to premature spine, hip, and wrist fractures, but orthopaedists already are seeing an increased incidence of stress fractures in these amenorrheic athletes. Other musculoskeletal problems also are more common in the female athlete; these problems include scoliosis in the spine, patellofemoral problems and anterior cruciate ligament injuries in the knee, and bunions and increased pronation in the foot. The biggest problem in the foot is related to the fact that most shoes for athletics are designed for men and have been scaled down but not adapted to the shape of the woman's foot.

This monograph presents the latest information on these and other issues concerning the female athlete.

CAROL C. TEITZ, MD

REFERENCES

1. Lopiano DA: Gender equity in sports, in Agostini R, Titus S (eds): *Medical and Orthopedic Issues of Active and Athletic Women.* Philadelphia, PA, Hanley & Belfus, 1994, pp 13-22.

2. Cann CE, Martin MC, Genant HK, et al: Decreased spinal mineral content in amenorrheic women. *JAMA* 1984;251:626-629.

3. Nattiv A, Yeager K, Drinkwater B, et al: The female athlete triad, in Agostini R, Titus S (eds): *Medical and Orthopedic Issues of Active and Athletic Women.* Philadelphia, PA, Hanley & Belfus, 1994, pp 169-174.

PREPARTICIPATION EVALUATION

SUZANNE M. TANNER, MD

The preparticipation evaluation is meant to enhance the health and safety of athletes. Although ideally the preparticipation evaluation is not intended as a substitute for the athlete's regular health maintenance examinations, it serves as the only annual medical examination for 78% of school-age athletes.[1] For these athletes, a preparticipation evaluation is required before participation in interscholastic and intercollegiate sports is allowed. In the adult woman, entry into certain community sports programs may require preparticipation evaluation and clearance. More commonly, a preparticipation evaluation is advised for women who want to begin an exercise program, particularly those women older than 40 years of age. In this group of women, the evaluation should consist of a complete medical history and physical examination, including a thorough musculoskeletal assessment. The type and intensity of exercise suggested might be affected by a history of cardiac or pulmonary problems, urinary incontinence, or musculoskeletal injury. Cardiac stress testing is recommended only for women older than 50 years of age who have risk factors for coronary artery disease, such as high low-density lipoprotein (LDL) cholesterol levels, an abnormal resting electrocardiogram (ECG), or a history of angina.[2] It is also recommended for younger women with a strong family history of coronary artery disease or sudden death. However, it is important to remember that cardiac stress testing is not a totally reliable predictor of acute coronary events.[3] Although the content of the preparticipation evaluation is identical in many areas for males and females, active women and girls require special attention in the areas of nutritional status, body composition, menstrual status, growth and development, and musculoskeletal examination.

OBJECTIVES OF THE EVALUATION

According to *Preparticipation Physical Evaluation,* a monograph developed by the American Orthopaedic Society for Sports Medicine[4] and other national organizations, the evaluation has three primary objectives. First, the evaluation is used to detect any condition that may limit an athlete's participation. If an athlete has seizures that are not well controlled with medication, for example, further evaluation and treatment are required before the athlete may participate in certain sports, such as swimming. Second, the evaluation should detect any condition that may limit an athlete's safe participation or may be potentially life-threatening or disabling. An incompletely healed or rehabilitated knee sprain is more likely to be reinjured. Third, the evaluation may help to meet legal and insurance requirements. Requirements for clearance of an athlete to participate in organized sports vary from state to state. Most states require that the evaluation be performed by a physician.[5]

The preparticipation physical evaluation also has several secondary objectives: to determine the general health of the athlete, to counsel the athlete on health maintenance issues, and to assess physical maturity, fitness, and performance.

The athlete can be counseled regarding proper nutrition, weight control, physical conditioning, seat belt use, drinking and driving, drug use, breast self-examination, contraception, and prevention of sexually transmitted diseases (Fig. 1).[6] Physical maturity may be assessed by examining the degree of development of breasts and pubic hair. Some argue that for contact and collision sports, grouping school-age participants according to physical maturity rather than chronologic age would lessen the risk of injury to less mature

Portions of this chapter were adapted from an earlier work by the author,
Preparticipation examination targeted for the female athlete. *Clin Sports Med* 1994;13:337-353.

HEALTH MAINTENANCE: LIFESTYLE QUESTIONNAIRE

Instructions to athlete:
Answer the following questions yourself.
Check the correct answer.

1. Do you wear your seat belt?	☐ often	☐ occasionally	☐ rarely	☐ never
2. Have you ever smoked?	☐ often	☐ occasionally	☐ rarely	☐ never
3. Have you ever drunk alcohol?	☐ often	☐ occasionally	☐ rarely	☐ never
4. Have you ever used drugs?	☐ often	☐ occasionally	☐ rarely	☐ never
5. Have you ever used anabolic steroids?	☐ often	☐ occasionally	☐ rarely	☐ never
6. How often do your parents or guardians drink alcohol or use drugs?	☐ often	☐ occasionally	☐ rarely	☐ never
7. Have you ever been sexually active?	☐ often	☐ occasionally	☐ rarely	☐ never

FIGURE 1

Lifestyle questionnaire. (Reproduced with permission from *Preparticipation Physical Evaluation,* ed 2. Minneapolis, MN, The Physician and Sportsmedicine, 1997.)

individuals. There are no data to support this claim, however.[4] Fitness and performance can be assessed through optional tests, such as measurement of strength, flexibility, power, speed, endurance, balance, and agility. Test results may be used to guide conditioning.

TIMING, FREQUENCY, AND FORMAT OF THE EVALUATION

Ideally, the preparticipation physical evaluation should be conducted at least 6 weeks before the start of practice. This allows time for evaluation and treatment of health disorders, rehabilitation following injuries,[4] and institution of conditioning programs.

Requirements for frequency of evaluations vary by state. Although the American Academy of Pediatrics recommends that a complete evaluation be performed biennially, with an interim history and limited examination in alternate years,[7] this approach is possible only if the athlete's previous health records are thorough and readily available. No specific recommendations are made for adults.[8]

The preparticipation evaluation may be conducted individually in the privacy of a physician's office or by mass screening using multiple stations. Office-based evaluation allows continuity of care, a quiet setting for performing the cardiovascular examination, greater willingness of patients to discuss personal and gynecologic concerns, and better communication with parents of school-age athletes. The advantages of the station format include use of specialized personnel, efficient completion of numerous examinations, opportunity for fitness testing, greater communication with the school athletic staff,[4] and possible involvement of athletic trainers or physical therapists in providing exercise instruction. A sample of stations for a mass-screening format is shown in Table 1.

TABLE 1

STATIONS FOR MASS-SCREENING PREPARTICIPATION EVALUATIONS

Stations	Possible Personnel
Required	
Registration	Ancillary staff
Height and weight	Ancillary staff
Blood pressure, pulse	Ancillary staff
Vision	Ancillary staff
Medical examination	Physician
Musculoskeletal examination	Physician
Clearance	Physician
Optional	
Nutrition	Dietitian
Dental	Dentist
Body composition	Nurse, athletic trainer, or physical therapist
Fitness tests (strength, flexibility, power, speed, endurance, balance and agility)	Athletic trainer, physical therapist, exercise physiologist, or coach

(Adapted with permission from *Preparticipation Physical Evaluation*, ed 2. Minneapolis, MN, The Physician and Sportsmedicine, 1997.)

MEDICAL HISTORY

The medical history is the foundation of the preparticipation evaluation. Between 63% and 74% of problems affecting athletes can be detected from a complete history.[1,9] In children and adolescents, the preparticipation questionnaire (Fig. 2) is best answered by the athlete and her parent(s)

because only 39% of histories given by athletes alone agree with those provided by parents.[1] Questions about drug use and sexual activity (Fig. 1) should be answered only by the athlete.

The preparticipation physical evaluation questionnaire saves time and ensures that major medical areas are screened. However, careful listening and verbal questioning by the examiner may be more revealing. Some athletes may be tempted always to answer "no" on the questionnaire because positive answers may mean disqualification from sports.

Athletes should be aware that drug testing, for both nonprescription and prescription drugs, may be required before or after participation in events sponsored by the National Collegiate Athletic Association (NCAA) and the International Olympic Committee (IOC). Positive tests for disallowed drugs may result in disqualification. Updated lists of drugs that are allowed or banned may be obtained by contacting the NCAA (1-913-339-1906) or the United States Olympic Committee Drug Hotline (1-800-233-0393).

A questionnaire (Fig. 3) may also be used to detect nutritional deficiencies, eating disorders, and menstrual abnormalities. A large discrepancy between the athlete's actual weight and the desired weight for height should raise suspicion of an eating disorder. Pathologic weight-control behavior is prevalent, occurring in 32% of collegiate female athletes.[10] However, athletes with anorexia nervosa or bulimia may deny using pathologic weight-control methods, such as self-induced vomiting and diuretics.

In females without eating disorders, inadequate consumption of protein, iron, and calcium are common, particularly in those who attempt to decrease fat intake by avoiding red meat. The recommended daily intake of protein for active women younger than 25 years of age, and for pregnant and lactating women, is 0.5 to 0.75 g/lb of body weight.[11] This is equivalent to 60 to 90 g of protein for a 120-lb woman, or one 4- to 6-oz serving of meat. For women older than 25 years of age who are neither pregnant nor lactating, the recommended daily intake of protein is 0.36 g/lb of body weight.[12] For vegetarians, protein can be obtained in beans, grains, and eggs. Soy proteins are nutritionally equivalent to animal protein. Sufficient iron can usually be obtained by eating red meat two or three times a week, but it also is found in dried beans, fruits, grains, and fortified

Preparticipation Physical Evaluation

DATE OF EXAM _____

Name _____ Sex _____ Age _____ Date of birth _____

Grade ____ School _____ Sport(s) _____

Address _____ Phone _____

Personal physician _____

In case of emergency, contact

Name _____ Relationship _____ Phone (H) _____ (W) _____

**Explain "Yes" answers below.
Circle questions you don't know the answers to.**

	Yes	No
1. Have you had a medical illness or injury since your last check up or sports physical?	☐	☐
Do you have an ongoing or chronic illness?	☐	☐
2. Have you ever been hospitalized overnight?	☐	☐
Have you ever had surgery?	☐	☐
3. Are you currently taking any prescription or nonprescription (over-the-counter) medications or pills or using an inhaler?	☐	☐
Have you ever taken any supplements or vitamins to help you gain or lose weight or improve your performance?	☐	☐
4. Do you have any allergies (for example, to pollen, medicine, food, or stinging insects)?	☐	☐
Have you ever had a rash or hives develop during or after exercise?	☐	☐
5. Have you ever passed out during or after exercise?	☐	☐
Have you ever been dizzy during or after exercise?	☐	☐
Have you ever had chest pain during or after exercise?	☐	☐
Do you get tired more quickly than your friends do during exercise?	☐	☐
Have you ever had racing of your heart or skipped heartbeats?	☐	☐
Have you had high blood pressure or high cholesterol?	☐	☐
Have you ever been told you have a heart murmur?	☐	☐
Has any family member or relative died of heart problems or of sudden death before age 50?	☐	☐
Have you had a severe viral infection (for example, myocarditis or mononucleosis) within the last month?	☐	☐
Has a physician ever denied or restricted your participation in sports for any heart problems?	☐	☐
6. Do you have any current skin problems (for example, itching, rashes, acne, warts, fungus, or blisters)?	☐	☐
7. Have you ever had a head injury or concussion?	☐	☐
Have you ever been knocked out, become unconscious, or lost your memory?	☐	☐
Have you ever had a seizure?	☐	☐
Do you have frequent or severe headaches?	☐	☐
Have you ever had numbness or tingling in your arms, hands, legs, or feet?	☐	☐
Have you ever had a stinger, burner, or pinched nerve?	☐	☐
8. Have you ever become ill from exercising in the heat?	☐	☐
9. Do you cough, wheeze, or have trouble breathing during or after activity?	☐	☐
Do you have asthma?	☐	☐
Do you have seasonal allergies that require medical treatment?	☐	☐

	Yes	No
10. Do you use any special protective or corrective equipment or devices that aren't usually used for your sport or position (for example, knee brace, special neck roll, foot orthotics, retainer on your teeth, hearing aid)?	☐	☐
11. Have you had any problems with your eyes or vision?	☐	☐
Do you wear glasses, contacts, or protective eyewear?	☐	☐
12. Have you ever had a sprain, strain, or swelling after injury?	☐	☐
Have you broken or fractured any bones or dislocated any joints?	☐	☐
Have you had any other problems with pain or swelling in muscles, tendons, bones, or joints?	☐	☐

If yes, check appropriate box and explain below.

☐ Head	☐ Elbow	☐ Hip
☐ Neck	☐ Forearm	☐ Thigh
☐ Back	☐ Wrist	☐ Knee
☐ Chest	☐ Hand	☐ Shin/calf
☐ Shoulder	☐ Finger	☐ Ankle
☐ Upper arm		☐ Foot

	Yes	No
13. Do you want to weigh more or less than you do now?	☐	☐
Do you lose weight regularly to meet weight requirements for your sport?	☐	☐
14. Do you feel stressed out?	☐	☐

15. Record the dates of your most recent immunizations (shots) for:

Tetanus _____ Measles _____

Hepatitis B _____ Chickenpox _____

FEMALES ONLY

16. When was your first menstrual period? _____

When was your most recent menstrual period? _____

How much time do you usually have from the start of one period to the start of another? _____

How many periods have you had in the last year? _____

What was the longest time between periods in the last year? _____

Explain "Yes" answers here: _____

_____

_____

_____

_____

_____

_____

_____

_____

I hereby state that, to the best of my knowledge, my answers to the above questions are complete and correct.

Signature of athlete _____ Signature of parent/guardian _____ Date _____

FIGURE 2

History questionnaire. (Reproduced with permission from *Preparticipation Physical Evaluation,* ed 2. Minneapolis, MN, The Physician and Sportsmedicine, 1997.)

HEALTH MAINTENANCE: NUTRITIONAL AND MENSTRUAL QUESTIONNAIRE FOR FEMALES

1. How much would you like to weigh? _____ lbs.

2. How many meals do you eat each day? _____

3. How many snacks do you eat each day? _____

4. List any foods you avoid. _____

_____

5. Have you ever used any of the following methods to lose weight?

	Yes	No
diet pills	☐	☐
vomiting	☐	☐
laxatives	☐	☐
diuretics (increase urine output)	☐	☐

6. Have you ever been diagnosed as having an eating disorder? _____

7. Do you have questions about nutrition or your weight? _____

8. At what age did your menstrual periods start? _____ years

9. When was your most recent menstrual period? _____

10. Approximately how many menstrual periods did you have during the last 12 months? _____

FIGURE 3

Nutritional and menstrual questionnaire. (Reproduced with permission from *Preparticipation Physical Evaluation,* ed 2. Minneapolis, MN, The Physician and Sportsmedicine, 1997.)

flour and cereal. Absorption of nonheme iron, the kind found in plant foods, is inhibited by caffeine and enhanced by ascorbic acid.[12]

Low calcium intake may predispose the athlete to poor bone mineralization. Teenagers, young adult women, and postmenopausal women should consume at least 1,500 mg of calcium per day. This may be provided by three to four servings of dairy products, such as low-fat milk or yogurt,[11] or calcium supplements, such as calcium carbonate or calcium citrate.[13]

A menstrual history is also critical. In addition to questions about intensity of menstrual flow and dysmenorrhea, the history should include the age of menarche, frequency and duration of menstrual periods, date of last menstrual period, and use of hormonal therapy. An athlete who has unusually heavy menstrual flow should be examined for anemia.[14] Antiprostaglandin medication, such as nonsteroidal anti-inflammatory drugs, may reduce dysmenorrhea that interferes with exercise.[14] The median age of menarche is 12.5 years for black American girls and 12.8 years for white American girls.[15,16] Women involved in intense sports competition may be relieved when they are not inconvenienced by menstrual periods. However, abnormal menses may have deleterious effects on the skeleton and should not be attributed to exercise alone.[17] Further workup is suggested for women with amenorrhea and those with irregular menses, cycles shorter than 25 days, or cycles longer than 35 days.[14,18]

Preparticipation Physical Evaluation

PHYSICAL EXAMINATION

Name ______________________________ **Date of birth** ______________

Height _______ **Weight** _______ **% Body fat (optional)** _______ **Pulse** _____ **BP** ___/___ (___/___ , ___/___)

Vision R 20/ ____ **L 20/** ____ **Corrected: Y N** **Pupils: Equal** ____ **Unequal** ____

	NORMAL	ABNORMAL FINDINGS	INITIALS*
MEDICAL			
Appearance			
Eyes/Ears/Nose/Throat			
Lymph Nodes			
Heart			
Pulses			
Lungs			
Abdomen			
Genitalia (males only)			
Skin			
MUSCULOSKELETAL			
Neck			
Back			
Shoulder/arm			
Elbow/forearm			
Wrist/hand			
Hip/thigh			
Knee			
Leg/ankle			
Foot			

* Station-based examination only

CLEARANCE

❑ **Cleared**

❑ **Cleared after completing evaluation/rehabilitation for:** ______________________________

❑ **Not cleared for:** ______________________ **Reason:** ______________________

Recommendations: ______________________________

Name of physician (print/type) ______________________________ **Date** __________

Address ______________________________ **Phone** __________

Signature of physician ______________________________, **MD or DO**

FIGURE 4

Physical examination record. (Reproduced with permission from *Preparticipation Physical Evaluation,* ed 2. Minneapolis, MN, The Physician and Sportsmedicine, 1997.)

PHYSICAL EXAMINATION

A physical examination record is provided in Figure 4. Special attention should be paid to body composition, growth and development, assessment of sexual maturity, pulmonary evaluation, cardiovascular status assessment, neurologic evaluation, and musculoskeletal examination.

BODY COMPOSITION

Measuring height and weight and comparing the results to growth charts may help identify athletes with a growth abnormality who require further evaluation.[4] If an athlete appears obese or too thin, adiposity may be estimated using skinfold calipers. Although it is impossible to make an exact prediction of an athlete's ideal weight in terms of promoting health, growth, and sports performance, an estimate may be generated using the following equations based on Figure 5:

Estimated ideal weight for an obese athlete =

$$\left(1- \frac{\text{actual body fat} - \text{desired \% body fat}}{100}\right) \times \text{current weight}$$

Estimated ideal weight for a thin athlete =

$$\left(1+ \frac{\text{actual body fat} - \text{desired \% body fat}}{100}\right) \times \text{current weight}$$

Example: A 21-year-old female volleyball player weighs 160 lb. Her percent body fat, as estimated from skinfold calipers, is 25%. Her ideal % body fat is 16%. Her estimated ideal weight is calculated:

$$\left(1- \frac{25-16}{100}\right) \times 160 = (1-0.09) \times 160 = (0.91) \times 160 = 146 \text{ lbs}$$

It should be emphasized strongly to the athlete that this weight goal is only an estimate. These equations may not apply to prepubertal athletes. For obese females, elimination of snacks and a decrease in fat intake may promote weight loss.

GROWTH AND DEVELOPMENT

In girls, puberty usually starts between 8 and 14 years of age and ends about 3 years later. The growth spurt usually begins at the onset of stage two sexual maturity in girls, peaks at stage three, and ends at stage five.[7] Girls may increase their

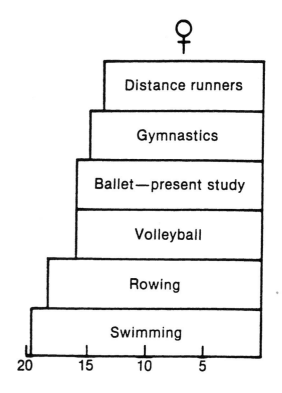

FIGURE 5

Body composition of female athletes (percent body weight as fat). (Reproduced with permission from Kirkendall DT, Calabrese LH: Physiological aspects of dance. *Clin Sports Med* 1983;2:533.)

height by about 20% during puberty,[14] but growth after menarche is limited to about 7.4 cm. Although menarche is the most commonly reported maturational event, it occurs relatively late in puberty, during stage four, as the growth rate is declining.[7,16]

ASSESSING SEXUAL MATURITY

Assessing the stage of sexual maturity in a female athlete helps determine whether a girl is suffering from primary amenorrhea. The examiner can then provide guidance about future physical development or the possible need for further endocrinologic evaluation.

Sexual maturity in young girls can be assessed by the examiner or by self-assessment of pubic hair and breast development. In one study, self-assessment using diagrams of the stages of sexual maturation (Fig. 6) correlated well with the rating of sexual maturation determined by an examining physician.[19]

A

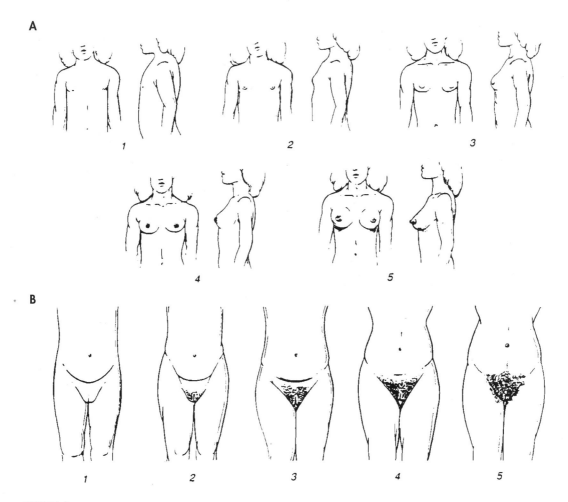

B

FIGURE 6

Stages of female sexual maturation. **Top** and **center,** Based on breast examination, stages are (1) prepubertal; no glandular tissue; (2) breast bud, small amount of glandular tissue; (3) breast mound and areola ernlarged, no contour separation; (4) breast enlarged, areola and papilla form mound projecting from breast contour; and (5) mature, areola part of breast contour. **Bottom,** Based on pelvic examination, stages are (1) no hair; (2) sparse, long, straight, lightly pigmented on labia majoria; (3) darker, beginning to curl, extend laterally; (4) coarse curly, abundant, less than adult; and (5) adult type and quantity, extending to medial thigh. (Reproduced with permission from Tanner SM: Preparticipation examination targeted for the female athlete. *Clin Sports Med* 1994;13:337-353.)

An additional although controversial reason for assessing sexual maturity in the adolescent athlete is to assign athletes to teams based on maturation level. Hypothetically, the risk of injury in contact sports might be decreased by grouping competitors on the basis of physical maturity rather than age. However, many sports organizations tend to group participants according to age, and strength does not correlate with sexual maturation stage as closely in girls as it does in boys.

PULMONARY EVALUATION

The athlete should be questioned about coughing after exercise, shortness of breath, and chest pain, which may be signs of exercise-induced asthma (EIA). This condition is underdiagnosed and undertreated. In childhood, the male:female incidence ratio is about 2:1, but by 30 years of age the ratio equalizes.[20] Wheezing is not always present. EIA need not sideline an athlete. Eleven percent of American athletes competing in the 1984

Olympic Games had signs and symptoms of EIA; of these athletes, 42% were female.[20] Swimming is the sport that usually is tolerated best by athletes with EIA. Warm-up and use of a beta-agonist inhaler prior to exercise may lessen symptoms.

Drugs allowed by the International Olympic Committee for treating asthma during Olympic competition include inhaled beta-2 agonists, cromolyn, and theophylline. However, written notification by the prescribing physician of the use of inhaled beta-2 agonists must be filed with the United States Olympic Committee prior to competition.

CARDIOVASCULAR EXAMINATION

Athletes with exercise-related syncope, palpitations, chest pain, and dyspnea or excessive fatigue should be identified and referred for cardiac evaluation.[21-23] A family history of sudden premature cardiac death, hypertrophic cardiomyopathy, Marfan syndrome, or premature coronary artery disease by 35 years of age also warrants further evaluation.[24]

The most common cause of sudden death in athletes younger than 35 years of age is congenital heart disease, such as hypertrophic cardiomyopathy. In older athletes, coronary artery disease is the most common cause,[25] although the risk of sudden death is lower for women than for men.[26] The murmur of hypertrophic cardiomyopathy, if present, tends to increase in intensity with Valsalva's maneuver.[27] Heart murmurs are common in adolescents and children, but any athlete with a significant murmur should have clearance deferred until further evaluation is completed.[4]

Mitral valve prolapse (MVP) is found in 5% of the general population compared with 17% of young women and girls.[28] The prevalence of MVP in athletes is not known, but more than 60% of adults with MVP are women. Patients with MVP range from asymptomatic (most common) to those with severe mitral regurgitation, infective endocarditis, cerebrovascular accidents, and sudden death. MVP may be part of a generalized connective tissue disorder such as Marfan syndrome. Still other patients have associated autonomic dysfunction and neuroendocrine abnormalities, such as increased serum levels of catecholamines.[28] These patients may complain of chest pain, dyspnea, palpitations, and even panic attacks. Ninety-two percent of individuals with MVP have a midsystolic click, with or without a late systolic murmur.[29] The click and murmur can be made to move closer to the first heart sound by asking the patient to sit or stand, thereby reducing left ventricular volume. Squatting increases left ventricular volume and will cause the murmur to decrease. Patients with these auscultatory findings should be referred for echocardiography. The echocardiogram can identify those patients who are at some risk of complications and who require further workup, counseling, and possible treatment. The vast majority of patients with MVP will be able to continue exercising without serious complications.[28] A task force on cardiovascular abnormalities in the athlete has published recommendations regarding eligibility for athletic competition based on various cardiac disorders.[23]

Athletes of any age with hypertension should be referred for further evaluation if the blood pressure is greater than 125/75 in an athlete younger than 10 years, or if it is greater than 135/85 in an athlete older than 10 years of age.[4,8]

NEUROLOGIC EXAMINATION

One of the most important parts of the neurologic examination is determining whether the athlete has a history of cerebral concussion, a transient alteration in mental function with or without loss of consciousness. This is a common injury in contact and collision sports, such as soccer and field hockey. The Colorado Medical Society Sports Medicine Committee developed guidelines for the management of concussion in athletes.[30] These guidelines, summarized in Table 2, may assist in determining clearance during the preparticipation evaluation. The examiner must exercise caution in allowing an athlete to return to a contact or collision sport because death has occurred from second-impact syndrome, a fatal brain swelling following minor head contact in players who have symptoms from a prior concussion.[31]

MUSCULOSKELETAL EXAMINATION

A 13-step musculoskeletal screening examination is presented in Figures 7-12 and Outline 1. A more thorough joint examination is indicated in the event of previous or current injuries to make sure that the injured part has been completely rehabilitated. Although most injuries are more specific to a sport than to a gender, several musculoskeletal problems are more prevalent in females, including scoliosis, patellofemoral pain, anterior cruciate ligament tears, bunions, and

TABLE 2

GRADING CONCUSSIONS IN SPORTS AND GUIDELINES FOR RETURN TO PLAY

Grading		Guidelines		
Severity	Signs/symptoms	First concussion	Second concussion	Third concussion
Grade I (mild)	Confusion without amnesia; no loss of consciousness	May return to play if asymptomatic[††] for at least 20 minutes	Terminate contest/practice; may return to play if asymptomatic[††] for at least 1 week	Terminate season; may return to play in 3 months if asymptomatic[††]
Grade II (moderate)	Confusion with amnesia[*]; no loss of consciousness[†]	Terminate contest/practice; may return to play if asymptomatic[††] for at least 1 week	Consider terminating season, but may return to play if asymptomatic[††] for 1 month	Terminate season; may return to play next season if asymptomatic[††]
Grade III (severe)	Loss of consciousness[†]	Terminate contest/practice and transport to hospital; may return to play 1 month after 2 consecutive asymptomatic[††] weeks; conditioning allowed after 1 asymptomatic[††] week	Terminate season; may return to play next season if asymptomatic[††]	Terminate season; strongly discourage return to contact/ collision sports

[*] Posttraumatic amnesia (amnesia for events following the impact) or more severe retrograde amnesia (amnesia for events preceding the impact).

[†] Some clinicians include "brief" loss of consciousness in Grade II and reserve "prolonged" loss of consciousness for Grade III. However, the definitions of "brief" and "prolonged" are not universally accepted.

[††] No headache, confusion, dizziness, impaired orientation, impaired concentration, or memory dysfunction during rest or exertion.

(Adapted with permission from the Colorado Medical Society: *Report of the Sports Medicine Committee: Guidelines for the Management of Concussion in Sports.* Denver, Colorado, Colorado Medical Society, 1991, revised.)

stress fractures. (These conditions are discussed elsewhere in this monograph.)

LABORATORY TESTS

Routine laboratory screening tests are no longer recommended for adolescent athletes.[4] Dipstick urinalysis has not been shown to help identify renal pathology in asymptomatic school-age subjects,[32,33] nor have a complete blood count, ferritin, sickle cell test, serum electrolytes, or lipid assay been proven to be of value in this population. Nevertheless, up to 9% of high school- and college-age female athletes have iron deficiency anemia. An additional 20% to 62% of female ath-letes in high school and college are relatively iron deficient as manifested by low ferritin levels; however, they have normal hematocrits.[34] Although it is unclear whether restoring iron stores to normal in those patients who are not anemic improves performance, the hemoglobin in some of these women with nonanemic iron deficiency increases when they are given iron supplements. However, checking ferritin levels is controversial.[34] In women 45 to 65 years of age, lipid and cholesterol screening may reveal profiles that raise concern for coronary artery disease. Treatment has been shown to decrease the incidence of coronary events.[8]

OUTLINE 1

THE MUSCULOSKELETAL SCREENING EXAMINATION

1. Athlete faces examiner: Note general body habitus, vertical alignment of head, trunk, and lower extremities. Are shoulders level? Is waist symmetrical? (Figure 7, **A** and **B**)

2. Athlete's back to examiner: Note symmetry of shoulders, scapulae, and waist crease. Note symmetry of space between arms and trunk. (Figure 7, **C** and **D**)

3. Athlete bends forward: Look for scoliosis, asymmetry of scapulae or ribs. Note spinal motion, hamstring tightness. (Figure 7, **E** and **F**)

4. Athlete's back to examiner and bends forward: Look for scoliosis, rib prominence. (Figure 7, **G** and **H**)

5. Athlete tries to touch chin to chest, look at ceiling, look over each shoulder, touch ear to shoulder. Note restricted range of motion. (Figure 8)

6. Athlete places hands behind head: Note full abduction and external rotation of shoulders, and full flexion of elbows. (Figure 9, **A** and **D**)

7. Athlete's back to examiner and tries to place thumbs as far up on spine as possible: Note restricted range of motion or asymmetry. (Figure 9, **B** and **E**)

8. Athlete faces examiner and abducts shoulders against resistance with elbows extended: Note weakness in abduction or inability to extend elbows. (Figure 9, **C** and **F**)

9. Athlete holds elbows at sides and pronates and supinates forearms: Note restricted range of motion. (Figure 10, **A, B, D** and **E**)

10. Athlete makes fist and resists adduction of fingers: Note weakness or restricted range of motion. (Figure 10, **C** and **F**)

11. Note alignment of knees and feet. Are patellae straight ahead? Is athlete knock kneed or bowlegged? Are arches high or low? Is quadriceps bulk symmetrical? (Figure 11, **A-C**)

12. Athlete rises to tiptoes and walks: Note inversion of heels and calf strength. Athlete walks on heels: Note weakness.(Figure 11, **D-F**)

13. Athlete squats and duck walks: Note full hip, knee, and ankle flexion or any weakness. (Figure 12)

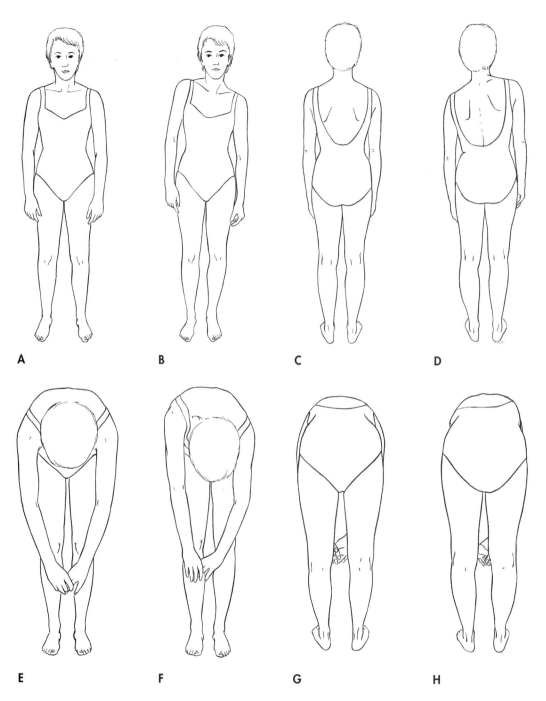

A   B   C   D

E   F   G   H

FIGURE 7

The musculoskeletal screening examination. Note general body habitus, vertical alignment of head, trunk, and lower extremities. Are shoulders level? Is waist symmetrical? **A,** normal; **B,** asymmetry of shoulders and space between arms and trunk. Note symmetry of shoulders, scapulae, waist crease, and of space between arms and trunk. **C,** normal; **D,** asymmetry of shoulders, scapulae, waist crease, and space between arms and trunk. Look for scoliosis, asymmetry of scapulae or ribs. Note spinal motion, hamstring tightness. **E,** normal; **F,** asymmetry of ribs. Look for scoliosis, rib prominence. **G,** normal; and **H,** asymmetry of ribs.

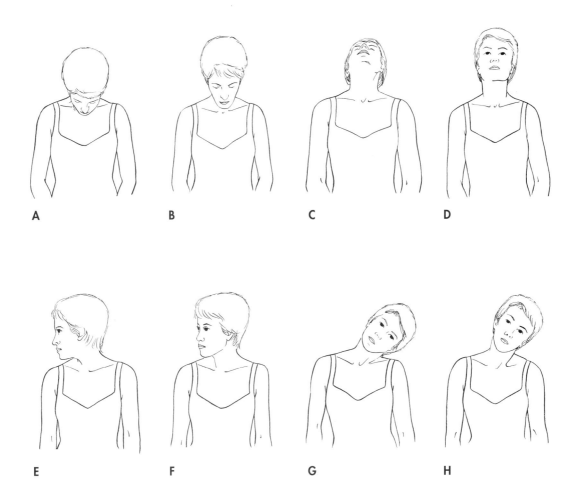

A   B   C   D

E   F   G   H

FIGURE 8

The musculoskeletal screening examination, continued. Athlete tries to touch chin to chest, look at ceiling, look over each shoulder, touch ear to shoulder. Note restricted range of motion. **A,** normal; **B,** restricted flexion; **C,** normal; **D,** restricted extension; **E,** normal; **F,** restricted sideward rotation; **G,** normal, and **H,** restricted lateral bending.

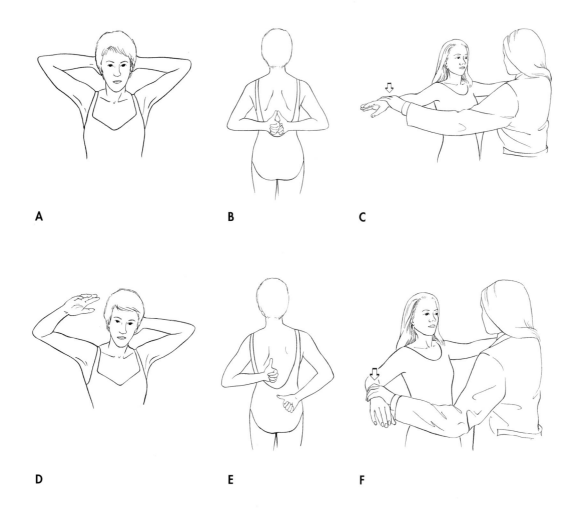

A   **B**   **C**

D   **E**   **F**

FIGURE 9

The musculoskeletal screening examination, continued. **A** and **D,** athlete places hands behind head. Note full abduction and external rotation of shoulders, and full flexion of elbows. **A-C,** normal; **B** and **E,** athlete tries to place thumbs as far up on spine as possible. Note restricted range of motion or asymmetry. **C** and **F,** athlete faces examiner and abducts shoulders against resistance with elbows extended. Note weakness in abduction or inability to extend elbows. **D,** lack of full external rotation; **E,** lack of full internal rotation of shoulder, flexion of elbow; and **F,** lack of shoulder abduction strength, full extension of elbow.

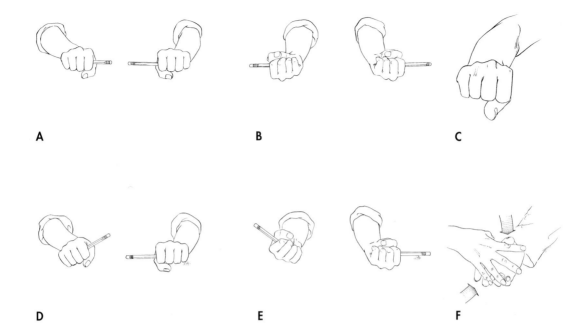

FIGURE 10
A, **B**, **D**, and **E**, athlete holds elbows at sides and pronates and supinates forearms. Note restricted range of motion.
C and **F**, athlete makes fist and resists adduction of fingers. Note weakness or restricted range of motion. **A-C**, normal;
D, asymmetrical pronation; **E**, asymmetrical supination; and **F**, athlete resists adduction of fingers.

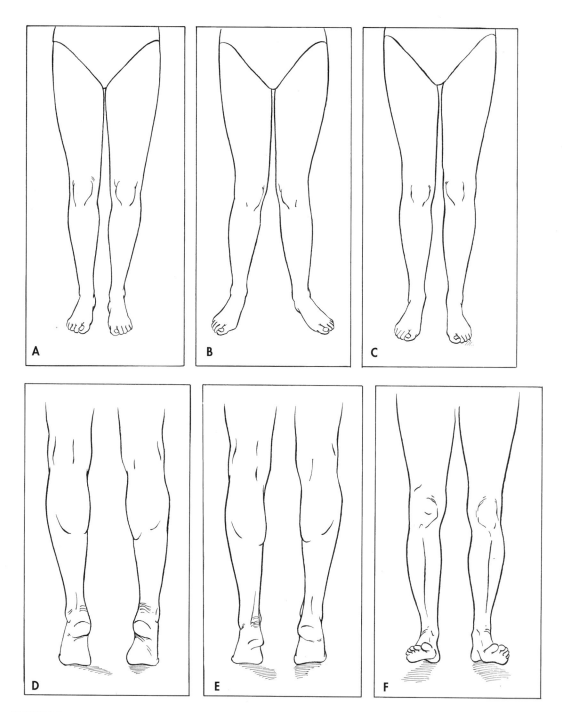

FIGURE 11

Note alignment of knees and feet. Are patellae straight ahead, is athlete knock kneed or bowlegged, are arches high or low, is quadriceps bulk symmetrical? **A,** normal; **B,** genu valgum (knock kneed and pronated feet); **C,** femoral anteversion (cross-eyed patellae) and pronated feet. Athlete rises to tiptoes and walks: Note inversion of heels and calf strength. Athlete walks on heels. Note weakness. **D,** normal; **E,** asymmetrical inversion of heels; and **F,** normal.

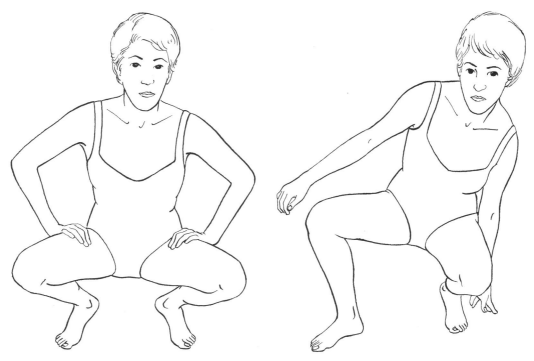

FIGURE 12
Athlete squats and duck walks. Note full hip, knee, and ankle flexion or any weakness. **Left,** normal; **right,** asymmetrical hip, knee, and ankle flexion.

CLEARANCE FOR PARTICIPATION

The most crucial question when conducting a preparticipation evaluation is, "is it safe for the athlete to participate in a sport?" The questions listed in Outline 2 should be answered when considering clearance for a medical or musculoskeletal problem.[4]

Clearance may be unrestricted, restricted until the athlete has completed an additional evaluation or rehabilitation, or not granted for any sport. Few athletes fail the examination, however. A review of five studies of preparticipation examinations performed on more than 17,500 male and female student athletes reveals that only 0.2% to 1.2% of participants fail the examination.[22,35-38]

The American Academy of Pediatrics provides guidance on determining whether or not it is safe to allow athletes with medical conditions to participate in sports (Table 3).[39] These guidelines pertain in adults as well.[40] When determining whether an athlete should be cleared for participation in a sport, or whether restriction from the activity is warranted, the risk that a certain sport

OUTLINE 2

CONSIDERATIONS FOR CLEARING THE ATHLETE FOR SPORTS PARTICIPATION

1. Does the problem place the athlete at increased risk of injury?

2. Is any other participant at risk of injury because of the problem?

3. Can the athlete safely participate with treatment (eg, medication, rehabilitation, bracing, or padding)?

4. Can limited participation be allowed while treatment is being initiated?

5. If clearance is denied only for certain activities, in what activities can the athlete safely participate?

will cause an injury or aggravate a medical condition should be considered. Sports can be classified in two ways: according to their potential for

TABLE 3

MEDICAL CONDITIONS AFFECTING SPORTS PARTICIPATION

Condition	May Participate?
Atlantoaxial instability (instability of the joint between cervical vertebrae 1 and 2) Explanation: Athlete needs evaluation to assess risk of spinal cord injury during sports participation.	Qualified Yes
Bleeding disorder Explanation: Athlete needs evaluation.	Qualified Yes
Cardiovascular diseases	
Carditis (inflammation of the heart) Explanation: Carditis may result in sudden death with exertion.	No
Hypertension (high blood pressure) Explanation: Those with significant essential (unexplained) hypertension should avoid weight and power lifting, body building, and strength training. Those with secondary hypertension (hypertension caused by a previously identified disease), or severe essential hypertension, need evaluation. Reference 42 defines significant and severe hypertension.	Qualified Yes
Congenital heart disease (structural heart defects present at birth) Explanation: Those with mild forms may participate fully; those with moderate or severe forms, or who have undergone surgery, need evaluation. Reference 43 defines mild, moderate, and severe disease for the common cardiac lesions.	Qualified Yes
Dysrhythmia (irregular heart rhythm) Explanation: Athlete needs evaluation because some types require therapy or make certain sports dangerous, or both.[43]	Qualified Yes
Mitral valve prolapse (abnormal heart valve) Explanation: Those with symptoms (chest pain, symptoms of possible dysrhythmia) or evidence of mitral regurgitation (leaking) on physical examination need evaluation. All others may participate fully.[43]	Qualified Yes
Heart murmur Explanation: If the murmur is innocent (does not indicate heart disease), full participation is permitted. Otherwise the athlete needs evaluation (see congenital heart disease and mitral valve prolapse above).	Qualified Yes
Cerebral palsy Explanation: Athlete needs evaluation.	Qualified Yes
Diabetes mellitus Explanation: All sports can be played with proper attention to diet, hydration, and insulin therapy. Particular attention is needed for activities that last 30 minutes or more.	Yes
Diarrhea Explanation: Unless disease is mild, no participation is permitted, because diarrhea may increase the risk of dehydration and heat illness. See "Fever" below.	Qualified No
Eating disorders	
Anorexia nervosa Bulimia nervosa Explanation: These patients need both medical and psychiatric assessment before participation.	Qualified Yes

TABLE 3 (CONTINUED)

Condition	May Participate?

Eyes

Functionally one-eyed athlete
Loss of an eye
Detached retina
Previous eye surgery or serious eye injury
    Explanation: A functionally one-eyed athlete has a best corrected visual acuity of < 20/40
    in the worse eye. These athletes would suffer significant disability if the better eye was
    seriously injured as would those with loss of an eye. Some athletes who have previously undergone
    eye surgery or had a serious eye injury may have an increased risk of injury because of weakened
    eye tissue. Availability of eye guards approved by the American Society for Testing Materials (ASTM)
    and other protective equipment may allow participation in most sports, but this must be judged on
    an individual basis.[44,45]   Qualified Yes

Fever
    Explanation: Fever can increase cardiopulmonary effort, reduce maximum exercise capacity,
    make heat illness more likely, and increase orthostatic hypotension during exercise.
    Fever may rarely accompany myocarditis or other infections that may make exercise dangerous.   No

Heat illness, history of
    Explanation: Because of the increased likelihood of recurrence, the athlete needs
    individual assessment to determine the presence of predisposing conditions and to
    arrange a prevention strategy.   Qualified Yes

HIV infection
    Explanation: Because of the apparent minimal risk to others, all sports may be played
    that the state of health allows. In all athletes, skin lesions should be properly covered,
    and athletic personnel should use universal precautions when handling blood or
    body fluids with visible blood.[46]   Yes

Kidney: absence of one
    Explanation: Athlete needs individual assessment for contact/collision and limited contact sports.   Qualified Yes

Liver: enlarged
    Explanation: If the liver is acutely enlarged, participation should be avoided because of risk of rupture.
    If the liver is chronically enlarged, individual assessment is needed before collision/contact
    or limited contact sports are played.   Qualified Yes

Malignancy
    Explanation: Athlete needs individual assessment.   Qualified Yes

Musculoskeletal disorders
    Explanation: Athlete needs individual assessment.   Qualified Yes

Neurologic

History of serious head or spine trauma, severe or repeated concussions, or craniotomy.[7,30]
    Explanation: Athlete needs individual assessment for collision/contact or limited contact sports,
    and also for noncontact sports if there are deficits in judgment or cognition. Recent research
    supports a conservative approach to management of concussion.[30]   Qualified Yes

Convulsive disorder, well controlled
    Explanation: Risk of convulsion during participation is minimal.   Yes

TABLE 3 (CONTINUED)

Condition	May Participate?
Convulsive disorder, poorly controlled Explanation: Athlete needs individual assessment for collision/contact or limited contact sports. Avoid the following noncontact sports: archery, riflery, swimming, weight or power lifting, strength training, or sports involving heights. In these sports, occurrence of a convulsion may be a risk to self or others.	Qualified Yes
Obesity Explanation: Because of the risk of heat illness, obese persons need careful acclimatization and hydration.	Qualified Yes
Organ transplant recipient Explanation: Athlete needs individual assessment.	Qualified Yes
Ovary: absence of one Explanation: Risk of severe injury to the remaining ovary is minimal.	Yes
Respiratory	
Pulmonary compromise including cystic fibrosis Explanation: Athlete needs individual assessment, but generally all sports may be played if oxygenation remains satisfactory during a graded exercise test. Patients with cystic fibrosis need acclimatization and good hydration to reduce the risk of heat illness.	Qualified Yes
Asthma Explanation: With proper medication and education, only athletes with the most severe asthma will have to modify their participation.	Yes
Acute upper respiratory infection Explanation: Upper respiratory obstruction may affect pulmonary function. Athlete needs individual assessment for all but mild disease. See "Fever" above.	Qualified Yes
Sickle cell disease Explanation: Athlete needs individual assessment. In general, if status of the illness permits, all but high exertion, collision/contact sports may be played. Overheating, dehydration, and chilling must be avoided.	Qualified Yes
Sickle cell trait Explanation: It is unlikely that individuals with sickle cell trait (AS) have an increased risk of sudden death or other medical problems during athletic participation except under the most extreme conditions of heat, humidity, and possibly increased altitude.[47] These individuals, like all athletes, should be carefully conditioned, acclimatized, and hydrated to reduce any possible risk.	Yes
Skin: boils, herpes simplex, impetigo, scabies, molluscum contagiosum Explanation: While the patient is contagious, participation in gymnastics with mats, martial arts, wrestling, or other collision/contact or limited contact sports is not allowed. Herpes simplex virus probably is not transmitted via mats.	Qualified Yes
Spleen, enlarged Explanation: Patients with acutely enlarged spleens should avoid all sports because of risk of rupture. Those with chronically enlarged spleens need individual assessment before playing collision/contact or limited contact sports.	Qualified Yes

(Reproduced with permission from the American Academy of Pediatrics, Committee on Sports Medicine and Fitness: Medical conditions affecting sports participation. *Pediatrics* 1994;94:757-760.)

injury from collision (Table 4), and according to their level of strenuousness and potential for aggravating pulmonary and cardiovascular problems (Table 5).[39]

TABLE 4

CLASSIFICATION OF SPORTS BY CONTACT

Contact/Collision	Limited Contact	Noncontact
Basketball	Baseball	Archery
Boxing*	Bicycling	Badminton
Diving	Cheerleading	Bodybuilding
Field hockey	Canoeing/kayaking (white water)	Bowling
Football	Fencing	Canoeing/kayaking (flat water)
Flag	Field events	Crew/rowing
Tackle	High jump	Curling
Ice hockey	Pole vault	Dancing
Lacrosse	Floor hockey	Field events
Martial arts	Gymnastics	Discus
Rodeo	Handball	Javelin
Rugby	Horseback riding	Shot put
Ski jumping	Racquetball	Golf
Soccer	Skating	Orienteering
Team handball	Ice	Power lifting
Water polo	In-line	Race walking
Wrestling	Roller	Riflery
	Skiing	Rope jumping
	Cross-country	Running
	Downhill	Sailing
	Water	Scuba diving
	Softball	Strength training
	Squash	Swimming
	Ultimate frisbee	Table tennis
	Volleyball	Tennis
	Windsurfing/surfing	Track
		Weight lifting

* Participation not recommended by the American Academy of Pediatrics. (Reproduced with permission from American Academy of Pediatrics, Committee on Sports Medicine and Fitness: Medical conditions affecting sports participation. *Pediatrics* 1994;94:757-760.)

TABLE 5

CLASSIFICATION OF SPORTS BY STRENUOUSNESS

High to Moderate Intensity		
High to Moderate Dynamic and Static Demands	High to Moderate Dynamic and Low Static Demands	High to Moderate Static and Low Dynamic Demands
Boxing*	Badminton	Archery
Crew/rowing	Baseball	Auto racing
Skiing	Basketball	Diving
Cross-country	Field hockey	Equestrian
Downhill	Lacrosse	Field events
Cycling	Orienteering	Jumping
Fencing	Ping-pong	Throwing
Football	Race walking	Gymnastics
Ice hockey	Racquetball	Karate or judo
Rugby	Soccer	Motorcycling
Running (sprint)	Squash	Rodeoing
Speed skating	Swimming	Sailing
Water polo	Tennis	Ski jumping
Wrestling	Volleyball	Water skiing
		Weight lifting

Low Intensity (Low Dynamic and Low Static Demands)

Bowling

Cricket

Curling

Golf

Riflery

* Participation not recommended by the American Academy of Pediatrics. (Reproduced with permission from American Academy of Pediatrics, Committee on Sports Medicine and Fitness: Medical conditions affecting sports participation. *Pediatrics* 1994;94:757-760.)

In female athletes, questions arise concerning protection of breasts and ovaries. Although breast contusions may occur, they are usually minor. Furthermore, there is no evidence that trauma predisposes to breast cancer.[41] Hence, recommendations for clearance or restriction (Outline 2) are identical for males and females, and no special restrictions for sports participation are necessary for female athletes with only one ovary.

REFERENCES

1. Risser WL, Hoffman HM, Bellah GG Jr: Frequency of preparticipation sports examinations in secondary school athletes: Are the University Interscholastic League guidelines appropriate? *Texas Med* 1985;81:35-39.

2. American College of Sports Medicine: *Guidelines for Exercise Testing and Prescription,* ed 4. Philadelphia, PA, Lea & Febiger, 1991.

3. Siscovick DS, Ekelund LG, Johnson JL, et al: Sensitivity of exercise electrocardiography for acute cardiac events during moderate and strenuous physical activity: The Lipid Research Clinics Coronary Primary Prevention Trial. *Arch Int Med* 1991;151:325-330.

4. *Preparticipation Physical Evaluation,* ed 2. Minneapolis, MN, The Physician and Sportsmedicine, 1997.

5. Feinstein RA, Soileau EJ, Daniel WA Jr: A national survey of preparticipation physical examination requirements. *Phys Sportsmed* 1988;16:51-59.

6. Krowchuk DP, Krowchuk HV, Hunter DM, et al: Parents' knowledge of the purposes and content of preparticipation physical examinations. *Arch Pediatr Adolesc Med* 1995;149:653-657.

7. Dyment PG (ed): *Sports Medicine: Health Care for Young Athletes,* ed 2. Elk Grove Village, IL, American Academy of Pediatrics, 1991.

8. US Preventive Services Task Force: *Guide to Clinical Preventive Services: Report of the U.S. Preventive Services Task Force,* ed 2. Baltimore, MD, Williams & Wilkins, 1996.

9. Goldberg B, Witman PA, Gleim GW, et al: Children's sports injuries: Are they avoidable? *Phys Sportsmed* 1979;7:93-101.

10. Rosen LW, McKeag DB, Hough DO, et al: Pathogenic weight-control behavior in female athletes. *Phys Sportsmed* 1986;14:79-86.

11. Clark N: Athletes with amenorrhea: Nutrition to the rescue. *Phys Sportsmed* 1993;21:45-48.

12. Vegetarian diets. *Harvard Women's Health Watch* 1996;3(5):2-3.

13. Guthrie M: Nutritional issues of exercise and performance, in Agostini R (ed): *Medical and Orthopaedic Issues of Active and Athletic Women.* Philadelphia, PA, Hanley & Belfus, 1994, pp 50-55.

14. Johnson MD: Tailoring the preparticipation exam to female athletes. *Phys Sportsmed* 1992;20:60-72.

15. Hale RW: Factors important to women engaged in vigorous physical activity, in Strauss RH (ed): *Sports Medicine,* ed 2. Philadelphia, PA, WB Saunders, 1991, pp 487-502.

16. Malina R: Growth, performance, activity and training during adolescence, in Shangold MM, Mirkin G (eds): *Women and Exercise: Physiology and Sports Medicine.* Philadelphia, PA, FA Davis, 1988, pp 120-128.

17. Nattiv A, Agostini R, Drinkwater B, et al: The female athlete triad: The inter-relatedness of disordered eating, amenorrhea, and osteoporosis. *Clin Sports Med* 1994;13:405-418.

18. Shangold MM: How I manage exercise-related menstrual disturbances. *Phys Sportsmed* 1986;14:113-120.

19. Duke PM, Litt IF, Gross RT: Adolescents' self-assessment of sexual maturation. *Pediatrics* 1980;66:918-920.

20. Voy RO: The U.S. Olympic Committee experience with exercise-induced bronchospasm, 1984. *Med Sci Sports Exerc* 1986;18:328-330.

21. Cheitlin MD: Evaluating athletes who have heart symptoms. *Phys Sportsmed* 1993;21:150-162.

22. Fahrenbach MC, Thompson PD: Minimizing the risk of exertional sudden death. *Your Patient and Fitness in Internal Medicine* 1993;7:6-12.

23. Maron BJ, Isner JM, McKenna WJ: 26th Bethesda Conference: Recommendations for determining eligibility for competition in athletes with cardiovascular abnormalities. Task Force 3: Hypertrophic cardiomyopathy, myocarditis, and other myopericardial diseases and mitral valve prolapse. *Med Sci Sports Exerc* 1994; 26:S261-S267.

24. Ades PA: Preventing sudden death: Cardiovascular screening of young athletes. *Phys Sportsmed* 1992;20:75-89.

25. Maron BJ, Epstein SE, Roberts WC: Causes of sudden death in competitive athletes. *J Am Coll Cardiol* 1986;7:204-214.

26. Cupples LA, Gagnon DR, Kannel WB: Long- and short-term risk of sudden coronary death. *Circulation* 1992;85(suppl 1):I11-I18.

27. Lembo NJ, Dell'Italia LJ, Crawford MH, et al: Bedside diagnosis of systolic murmurs. *N Engl J Med* 1988;318:1572-1578.

28. Joy E: Mitral valve prolapse in active patients: Recognition, treatment, and exercise recommendations. *Phys Sportsmed* 1996;24:78-86.

29. Washington RL: Mitral valve prolapse in active youth. *Phys Sportsmed* 1993;21:136-144.

30. Colorado Medical Society, Report of the Sports Medicine Committee: Guidelines for the management of concussion in sports (revised). Denver, CO, Colorado Medical Society, 1991.

31. Kelly JP, Nichols JS, Filley CM, et al: Concussion in sports: Guidelines for the prevention of catastrophic outcome. *JAMA* 1991;266:2867-2869.

32. Dodge WF, West EF, Smith EH, et al: Proteinuria and hematuria in schoolchildren: Epidemiology and early natural history. *J Pediatr* 1976; 88:327-347.

33. Vehaskari VM, Rapola J: Isolated proteinuria: Analysis of a school-age population. *J Pediatr* 1982;101:661-668.

34. Harris SS: Exercise-related anemias, in Agostini R (ed): *Medical and Orthopaedic Issues of Active and Athletic Women.* Philadelphia, PA, Hanley & Belfus, 1994, pp 270-275.

35. Tennant FS Jr, Sorenson K, Day CM: Benefits of preparticipation sports examinations. *J Fam Pract* 1981;13:287-288.

36. Linder CW, Durant RH, Seklecki RM, et al: Preparticipation health screening of young athletes: Results of 1268 examinations. *Am J Sports Med* 1981;9:187-193.

37. Thompson TR, Andrish JT, Bergfeld JA: A prospective study of preparticipation sports examinations of 2,670 young athletes: Method and results. *Cleve Clin Q* 1982;49:225-233.

38. Magnes SA, Henderson JM, Hunter SC: What conditions limit sports participation? Experience with 10,540 athletes. *Phys Sportsmed* 1992;20:143-158.

39. American Academy of Pediatrics Committee on Sports Medicine and Fitness: Medical conditions affecting sports participation. *Pediatrics* 1994; 94:757-760.

40. Maron BJ, Brown RW, McGrew CA, et al: Ethical, legal and practical considerations affecting medical decision-making in competitive athletes. *J Am Coll Cardiol* 1994;24:854-860.

41. Roy S, Irvin R: The female athlete, in Roy S, Irvin R (eds): *Sports Medicine: Prevention, Evaluation, Management, and Rehabilitiation.* Englewood Cliffs, NJ, Prentice-Hall, 1983, pp 457-467.

42. National Heart, Lung, Blood Institute: Report of the Second Task Force on Blood Pressure Control in Children–1987. *Pediatrics* 1987; 79:1-25.

43. Sixteenth Bethesda Conference: Cardiovascular abnormalities in the athlete: Recommendations regarding eligibility for competition. *J Am Coll Cardiol* 1985;6:1189-1190.

44. Dorsen PJ: Should athletes with one eye, kidney, or testicle play contact sports? *Phys Sportsmed* 1986;14:130-138.

45. Vinger PF: The one-eyed athlete. *Phys Sportsmed* 1987;15;48-52.

46. American Academy of Pediatrics, Committee on Sports Medicine Fitness: Human immunodeficiency virus [acquired immunodeficiency syndrome (AIDS) virus] in the athletic setting. *Pediatrics* 1991;88:640-641.

47. Pearson HA: Sickle cell trait and competitive athletics: Is there a risk? *Pediatrics* 1989; 83:613-614.

THE SPINE

SERENA S. HU, MD AND CAROL C. TEITZ, MD

Back problems in the female athlete include scoliosis, spondylolysis, muscle strains, sacroiliitis, and lumbar disk herniation. Their prevalence differs as a function of the age of the athlete. In the adolescent, spondylolysis and muscle strains are the most common causes of back pain. Scoliosis is also a problem in this age group, but does not present with pain. In the mature athlete, the physician must consider fractures and disk herniation in addition to strains and sacroiliac pathology. Back pain can also be referred from the uterus; thus gynecologic problems should be in the differential diagnosis of the female athlete presenting with low back pain.

SPONDYLOLYSIS AND SPONDYLOLISTHESIS

A young female gymnast, diver, or ballerina presenting with unilateral low back pain should be considered to have a spondylolysis until proven otherwise. In 1995, Micheli and Wood[1] reported that 62% of 100 athletes presenting with back pain were found to have a problem in the posterior elements of the spine. Ultimately, 47% were found to have spondylolysis.[1] In data from the 1996 NCAA Injury Surveillance System, the rate of low back injuries in female gymnasts was 1.06 per 1,000 athletic exposures compared with 0.09 per 1,000 athletic exposures in males.[2] Although spondylolysis is present in about 5% to 6% of the Caucasian population older than 6 years of age,[3] it is found in 11% to 15% of gymnasts, divers, and ballerinas.[4,5] These sports have in common hyperlordotic positioning of the spine. The repeated hyperlordosis associated with these sports is thought to produce recurrent bending stresses across the pars interarticularis, ultimately leading to a fatigue fracture.[6] Female gymnasts spend more time with their spines in hyperextension during floor exercise and balance beam (Fig. 13)

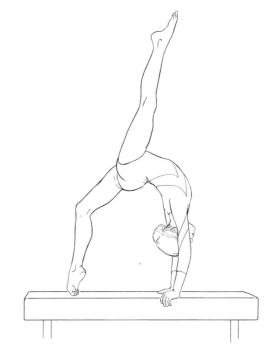

FIGURE 13
Spine hyperextension in the female gymnast.

than do male gymnasts, who emphasize strength more than flexibility. Furthermore, many elite female gymnasts are amenorrheic. Amenorrhea has been associated with an increased incidence of stress fractures in general (see "The Female Athlete Triad") and may contribute to fracture of the pars. In ballerinas as well, there is frequent hyperlordotic positioning of the trunk, which is seen in the most extreme example with high arabesque (Fig. 14). Dancers also have a high incidence of amenorrhea, which has been associated with stress fractures in their population as well.[7]

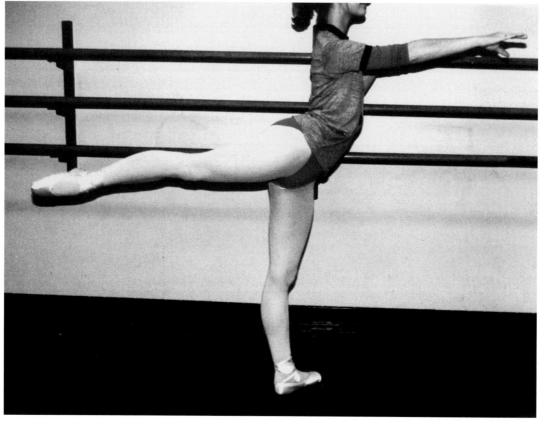

FIGURE 14

An arabesque can produce hyperlordosis of the lumbar spine. (Reproduced with permission from Teitz CC: Sports medicine concerns in dance and gymnastics. *Clin Sports Med* 1983;2:571-593.)

HISTORY AND PHYSICAL EXAMINATION

Ballerinas and gymnasts with a unilateral spondylolysis present with ipsilateral lumbar pain that usually does not radiate. The pain is typically insidious in onset, although there may be a history of a low-grade ache for some time followed by a recent sudden increase. The pain is made worse by hyperextension of the spine. The patient also may have noted recent hamstring tightness.

On physical examination, the physician finds tenderness to palpation at the level of the involved pars, just lateral to the midline. Muscle spasm, which produces a functional scoliosis, may be present. Pain can be reproduced by asking the patient to lean back while standing on the leg of the asymptomatic side and lifting the leg of the symptomatic side to the back. Prone hyperextension may also induce pain. The supine straight leg raising test does not usually produce any nerve root irritation, but may reveal hamstring tightness.[8]

The physician must remember that 90° of straight leg raising in these athletes is abnormally low, because gymnasts and dancers generally exhibit ligamentous laxity. They should be asked about their previous levels of flexibility.

ADDITIONAL STUDIES

Oblique radiographs of the lumbar spine will usually reveal a spondylolysis, whereas lateral views will reveal bilateral spondylolysis and spondylolisthesis. Pars defects can present as lucencies or sclerosis on the oblique radiograph of the lumbar spine (Fig. 15).[9] Computed tomography (CT) scans can help determine whether a pars defect is complete.[10] However, when lysis is suspected but not seen on radiographs, technetium diphosphonate bone scan should be

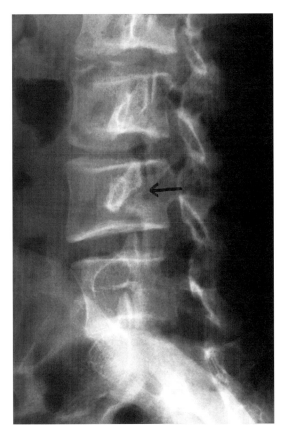

FIGURE 15
Spondylolysis on plain radiograph.

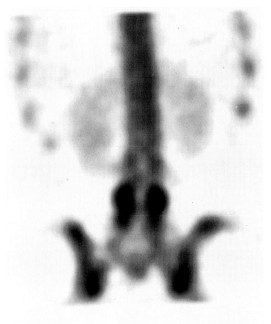

FIGURE 16
Spondylolysis on SPECT scan.

done.[11,12] The single photon emission computed tomography (SPECT) scan is more sensitive than traditional bone scan for localization of the uptake to the pars region (Fig. 16).[13] (Certainly a positive bone scan and a negative radiograph should also make the physician consider infection or osteoid osteoma. If the pain is not exacerbated by positioning or is present at rest, the physician should consider a diagnosis other than spondylolysis.) When lysis is visible on a radiograph, bone scan is still useful because it can determine whether the lysis is recent. If there is increased uptake on the scan and the history is consistent with recent trauma or overuse, the fracture is fresh and, in young patients, has some potential to heal with bracing. In patients with spondylolisthesis, lateral radiographs of the standing patient should be taken to determine percent slip and slip angle. The slip angle is mea-

sured between a line along the inferior border of L5 and a line perpendicular to the posterior border of the sacrum.[14] A normal angle is 0° (Fig. 17).

TREATMENT

The goals of treatment for an acute fracture are fracture healing and return to sports. The patient should be treated using a lumbosacral orthosis (LSO) that decreases lumbar lordosis.[15,16] Dancers are able to continue in class while wearing a brace. Gymnasts may be able to continue to practice on uneven parallel bars while wearing a brace. They also may be able to do balance beam and floor activities that are not limited by the brace. Brace use should continue until there is radiographic evidence of healing or until the bone scan does not show increased uptake. This typically takes 6 months, but may take longer. Healing has been described in 25% of these patients, although 78% obtained excellent clinical relief and returned to full activities.[16] Successful return to sports at the previous level of proficiency is more likely when the diagnosis of spondylolysis is made before radiographic lysis has occurred, and brace treatment is begun early.

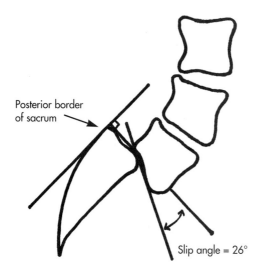

Posterior border
of sacrum

Slip angle = 26°

FIGURE 17
The slip angle. A line is drawn along the posterior aspect of
the sacrum and a perpendicular line to this is then drawn.
The angle between the perpendicular line and a line drawn
along the inferior border of L5 is the slip angle. In the example shown, the slip angle is 26°.

In the patient with an established lysis, the
goal is not healing of the fracture but rather
reduction of symptoms and return to sports.
These patients should be started on rehabilitation,
using a lumbosacral corset when necessary to
decrease pain. A similar rehabilitation program
can be used in the patient who is being treated in
a brace. Patients can return to sports when comfortable. They should initially avoid all maneuvers
that hyperextend the spine. Patients whose symptoms recur must decide whether to stop the exacerbating activity or to consider surgical treatment.

Horizontal translation between the vertebral
body with the pars defect and the vertebra below
is termed spondylolisthesis. Progression of
spondylolisthesis is more likely in females than
males[17] and is most likely to occur before the age
of 15 years. Slip angle is an important prognostic
indicator. Progression is more likely in patients
with slip angles greater than 55°.[14]

Patients with spondylolisthesis of 25% or less
often are able to return to sports when they are
asymptomatic after a brief period of rest followed
by rehabilitation.[18] Corsets are often helpful ini-

tially during the rest period, but the athlete must
understand that her abdominal and spine musculature will weaken with chronic brace wear.
Lateral radiographs should be repeated at
6-month intervals until skeletal maturity to make
sure that slippage is not increasing. For patients
with slips between 25% and 50%, activities that
do not hyperextend the lumbar spine are permitted.[19,20] Skeletally immature patients with slips
greater than 50% are at significant risk for slip
progression, and surgical fusion should be recommended. These patients typically are not able
to continue participation in dance or gymnastics.

Rehabilitation must concentrate on returning
the lumbar spine from a hyperlordotic position to
a normal amount of lumbar lordosis. Good trunk
control is key for both gymnasts and dancers,
particularly when they must balance on one leg.
In gymnasts, back bends, back walkovers, and so
forth tend to stretch the abdominal muscles.
Dancers, in an attempt to gain increased turnout,
often tip the pelvis forward, thereby loosening
the iliofemoral ligaments. Over time the anterior
inclination of the pelvis produces increased lordosis with stretched-out abdominals and tight hip
flexors. Moreover, in the adolescent, growth
spurts can produce quadriceps tightness and
tightness of the lumbodorsal fascia, which contribute to the hyperlordotic position of the pelvis.
Weakness of the iliopsoas muscles can also contribute to hyperlordosis because the iliopsoas
pulls on the lumbar spine when the thigh is
flexed in the nonweightbearing position (Fig. 18).
Therefore, stretching should be concentrated on
the rectus femoris and lumbodorsal fascia to allow
the pelvis to assume a more vertical position.

Abdominal strengthening should include the
rectus abdominis, abdominal obliques, and iliopsoas muscles. The iliopsoas can be strengthened
by performing straight legged hip flexion and
extension exercises in the supine position under
supervision of a therapist so that care is taken to
stabilize the lumbar spine and to make sure the
rectus femoris is not being recruited inadvertently.
Stretching the iliopsoas will also decrease hyperlordotic posturing. Use of the Pilates Reformer™
has proved very useful for these athletes.
The reformer allows strengthening of various
trunk and lower extremity muscles while controlling the position of the spine. Pilates exercises are
also useful in eliminating much of the gravitational pull while working on proper positioning of the

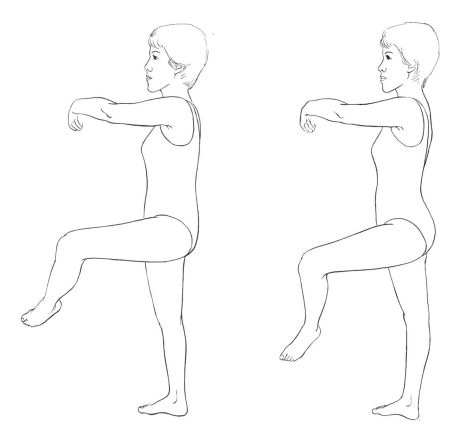

FIGURE 18
Hip flexion can increase lumbar lordosis in a dancer with a weak iliopsoas muscle. **Left,** normal; **right,** increased lordosis.

trunk and lower extremities during maneuvers that simulate what is necessary during sport or dance (Fig. 19).[21]

Patients whose symptoms are refractory to nonsurgical treatment and skeletally mature patients with a slip greater than 50% should be considered for surgical stabilization. Because spondylolisthesis most commonly occurs at L5–S1, stabilization is typically accomplished with a bilateral, lateral, single-level fusion.[22] When the slip is greater than 50%, however, the fusion bed is placed under tension and many advocate inclusion of L4 as well.[22] Overall fusion rates for this procedure are reported at 83% to 95%, with clinical results reported at 75% to 100% good to excellent.[23,24]

A young patient with pars defects at a level other than L5 and minimal or no slippage may be considered for a pars repair.[25-27] Repair can be accomplished by wiring the transverse processes to the spinous process or by placing a screw in the pedicle and then wiring the screw to the spinous process. The pars defects are cleaned and bone grafted.[28] Ninety percent of patients younger than 25 years of age with normal disks and facets and less than 1 to 2 mm of slippage can be expected to heal with good results.[25-28]

The hamstring tightness generally resolves, but may take 18 months to do so after fusion.[29] The majority of young patients with a successful fusion can return to sports as desired. However, these patients will lose a few degrees of motion. This loss may make return to gymnastics and dance more difficult than return to other sports. In addition, because it takes about 6 months for the fusion to mature and an additional 6 months to return to sport, gymnasts may lose the competitive edge in their peer group.

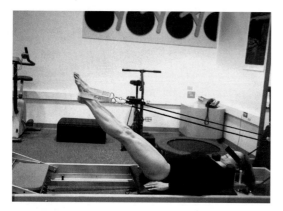

FIGURE 19
Use of the Pilates Reformer™ to strengthen trunk and lower extremity muscles.

SCOLIOSIS

Idiopathic scoliosis is more common in the adolescent female than male.[30,31] Its prevalence is even higher among ballerinas.[32] Idiopathic scoliosis occurs in 1% to 3% of the general population and in 3.9% of Caucasian girls. Warren and associates[32] found scoliosis in 24% of 75 Caucasian professional dancers whose mean age was 24.3 years, with a range from 18 to 36 years. The prevalence rose with increasing menarchal age. Eighty-three percent of dancers with scoliosis had delayed menarche (≥ 14 years) compared with 54% of dancers without scoliosis. Also, dancers with scoliosis had a slightly higher prevalence of secondary amenorrhea (44% versus 31%) and a significantly longer duration of amenorrhea (11.4 versus 4.1 months). Furthermore, the dancers with scoliosis and amenorrhea were significantly taller (171.2 cm versus 168.4 cm). The incidence of scoliosis in the families of the dancers with scoliosis was 28%, whereas the incidence in the families of the other dancers was 4%. Despite the fact that the subjects were no longer growing in height, two of the patients who had spinal radiograph evaluations for scoliosis had no fusion of the iliac apophyses at 19 years of age. The mean degree of curvature was 16.6° ± 8.5° (range 10° to 30°).[32] Although delayed puberty is a known risk factor for scoliosis, the frequency in the study group was thought to be above the expected frequency based on menarcheal age alone. Instead, the high prevalence was thought to be due to a combination of heredity, delayed maturation, and increased height.[32]

HISTORY AND PHYSICAL EXAMINATION

Young women with scoliosis are not symptomatic. However, during the preparticipation physical examination, the physician should examine the female athlete for this problem and be aware of the increased prevalence in dancers. In addition, the adolescent athlete should be asked about her menstrual history and about scoliosis in her immediate family.[33] Evaluation should include careful examination of the back, with the examiner looking for shoulder or pelvic obliquity, prominence of the scapula, or asymmetry of the waist, any of which suggest spinal curvature.

ADDITIONAL STUDIES

When scoliosis is suspected, an anteroposterior radiograph of the entire spine should be obtained in the standing patient. Degree of curvature should be determined by the Cobb method, measuring the angle between the end plates of the vertebrae maximally tilted into the concavity of the curve.

TREATMENT

The risk of curve progression is higher in patients who are premenarcheal and who have larger curves. Patients with curves less than 20° can be followed with clinical and radiographic examinations at 4- to 6-month intervals during the growth years.[34] Patients with curves greater than 20° and significant remaining skeletal growth and those whose curves have progressed more than 5° should be braced.[35]

Adolescent idiopathic curves where the apical vertebra is T8 or below can be managed with an underarm thoracolumbosacral orthosis (TLSO). In patients 10 to 15 years of age having thoracic curves measuring 25° to 35° with the apex between T8 and L1, brace management has been shown to be more effective than observation or electrical stimulation in preventing curve progression.[35] Thoracolumbar and lumbar curves (apex T11 or below) can be treated using a lumbosacral orthosis (LSO; Boston brace). Difficult-to-manage curves or curves with higher apices occasionally require a cervicothoracolumbosacral orthosis (CTLSO; Milwaukee brace). However, this brace is not acceptable to many preadolescent girls. Patients are permitted to be out of their braces a few hours a day to participate in sports. Braced patients should have follow-up radiographs at 4- to 6-month intervals during growth. Surgeons differ as to whether the follow-up radiographs should be taken with the patient in or out of the brace. When curves progress despite brace treatment, the brace is modified or surgical treatment is recommended, depending on the age of the patient and the size and location of the curve. Because brace wear may increase thoracic lordosis, it is important to consider the patient's sagittal alignment in order to avoid exacerbating one deformity while correcting another.

Patients and parents should be advised that although correction in the brace can be excellent, the long-term result of brace wear, at best, is arresting progression of the curve, rather than correcting it. Ideally, braces should be worn full time (bathing excepted). However, young athletic patients may remove their braces for several hours per day in order to participate in sports. Many dance activities can be carried out in an LSO, although it cannot be worn during performance. Exercise during the years of brace wear may actually prevent the muscle fatigue that often occurs when patients are weaned from their braces at skeletal maturity. Curves greater than 40° in adolescents generally require surgical treatment.

The majority of adolescents with progressive curves or curves greater than 40° can be satisfactorily treated with posterior spinal fusion.[36] Advances in instrumentation, with segmental attachment to the spine, have made it possible to eliminate or minimize bracing after surgical correction of thoracic curves in compliant young patients.[37,38] For primary lumbar or thoracolumbar curves, anterior release and fusion is the preferred option when no local kyphosis is present. Added correction is obtained by performing an anterior diskectomy and release.[39-41] Anterior fusion with instrumentation may permit correction of the curve while saving segments. For young athletic patients, this is a desirable goal. On the other hand, the retroperitoneal or thoracoabdominal scar is cosmetically less acceptable than a posterior midline scar. The surgeon must take care to maintain lumbar lordosis to avoid the later development of a disabling flatback syndrome.[42]

Beginning about 3 months postoperatively, patients in their teens and early 20s are gradually permitted to increase their sports activities. Swimming is permitted 6 to 12 weeks after surgery, depending on surgeon preference, patient comfort, and the levels fused. Stationary bicycling is permitted at the same time; road bicycling is generally discouraged until 3 or 4 months after surgery. Other sports may be permitted at 6 months after spinal fusion, although many surgeons forbid contact sports or running for a year after surgery. These time periods, of course, vary depending on the surgeon, quality of fixation, radiographic evidence of fusion, patient compliance, and the intensity of the patient's involvement in athletics. The majority of patients may return to all recreational activities by 1 year after surgery. Highly competitive athletes should be advised that spinal fusion will limit spinal motion. How this will affect performance is not predictable. For elite athletes in whom flexibility is crucial (gymnasts, dancers, divers), spinal fusion is likely to preclude performance at a highly competitive level. In some cases, surgical fusion can be delayed until completion of a patient's college athletic career, using periodic radiographs to ensure that the scoliosis is not progressing rapidly. Spinal fusion places additional stresses on the remaining motion segments. Therefore, patients should be advised that sports, such as running, that involve repetitive loading are particularly likely to increase stresses in the disks and facet joints adjacent to the fusion and predispose them to degeneration.

STRAINS

Overuse muscle strains of the lumbar erector spinae muscles are common in athletes who take part in sports, such as golf, soccer, softball, and modern dance, that require repeated rotation of the spine. Rowers using poor technique, in particular, using their backs instead of their thighs, also strain their backs. This is more likely to occur in women who are rowing in shells built for men, particularly when the seats do not fit. Micheli[43] also reported "mechanical back pain" occurring during periods of rapid growth and resulting from bony overgrowth overtaking ligamentous growth. This overgrowth was believed to lead to tight lumbodorsal fascia and hamstrings, with posterior decompensation of the torso over the pelvis and weak abdominal muscles, making strain of the shortened posterior musculature more likely.

HISTORY AND PHYSICAL EXAMINATION

The female athlete with a lumbar muscle strain usually presents after a specific incident in which she noticed mild back pain. The following day, her back is more painful and her range of motion restricted. The pain may be unilateral or bilateral and usually has no radicular component. Occasionally, the injury that causes the strain can also create swelling around the nerve roots producing pain in the femoral or sciatic nerve distributions. Motion aggravates the pain but Valsalva's maneuvers do not.

Muscle spasm is common, and the patient may walk listing to one side splinting the involved musculature. The involved muscles will be tender to palpation. The diagnosis often involves excluding other causes for back pain and spasm. In contrast to the pain from spondylolysis, the pain from a muscle strain is usually relieved by extension of the spine, but may be made worse by flexion. Dysrhythmia when returning from the forward flexed position is common. In contrast to the patient with these findings resulting from disk disease, straight leg raising tests are usually pain free, and the neurologic examination will be normal. There will be no aggravation of pain with Patrick's test.

As long as there is no bony tenderness, no night pain, and no systemic symptoms to suggest other diagnoses, no radiographs are required.

TREATMENT

The treatment is designed to decrease the spasm present following a strain. The spasm usually results from an inflammatory reaction to a microscopic tear in the muscle. Muscle spasm can be decreased either by applying heat, which will cause the muscle to relax, or applying ice massage, which also will cause relaxation by temporarily decreasing the nerve input to the muscle. After heat is used, there is a tendency for the muscle to go back into spasm as it cools to room temperature. After ice massage is used, the muscle usually stays relaxed as it warms to room temperature. Nonsteroidal anti-inflammatory drugs are helpful for pain relief and for decreasing the inflammatory reaction to the injury.

Transcutaneous electric nerve stimulation may be used if muscle spasm persists. The athlete usually should refrain from sports for a few days, while carrying on with supine knee-to-chest curls, which stretch the posterior musculature, and

extensor strengthening exercises. Early on these may be limited to hip lifting[44] (Fig. 20). To maintain abdominal strength without flexing the spine, the athlete can lie supine in the bent-knee position and push with straight arms against the anterior thighs. This exercise may be more comfortable than posterior pelvic tilt in the acute phase of lumbar strain. Prone extension exercises[45,46] that strengthen the musculature, and sport-specific stabilization exercises are added after acute pain has subsided. Pilates equipment is also useful in restoring trunk strength without gravitational loading.[21] Stretching and strengthening may also be required in hip flexors, hamstrings, tensor fascia lata muscles, and abdominal oblique muscles.

SACROILIAC PAIN

Sacroiliac pain is especially common in runners with a leg-length discrepancy greater than one half inch or in those running on a grade with a functional leg-length discrepancy. A true or functional leg-length discrepancy leads to shear stress in the sacroiliac joints.[47] Although this may be true in the male athlete as well, in women the pain should be differentiated from sacral pain secondary to menstrual cramps or uterine problems, such as fibroids in middle-aged women. Sacroiliitis is also a common feature of the seronegative spondyloarthropathies. Although these are traditionally diagnosed in males, they are indeed present in females[48] and are underdiagnosed. In the pregnant athlete, sacroiliac pain occurs as the result of loosening of ligaments and pelvic instability, particularly in the third trimester.[49]

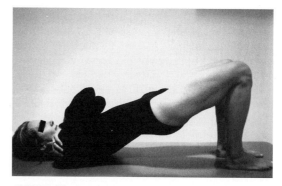

FIGURE 20
Hip lifting to strengthen extensor musculature.

The sacroiliac joint is a large, relatively immobile synovial joint that is poorly understood. It is stabilized by the joint capsule and the sacroiliac ligaments, and it is innervated variably. Pain from this joint may be localized or referred into the lower extremity.[50] The motion that occurs in the sacroiliac joint is disputed but may include rotation about the x-axis and translation about the z-axis. The joint is susceptible to axial compression and torsion; thus, forward bending, lifting, and twisting place stresses across the joint. Commonly reported mechanisms of injury are jumping, or landing hard on one leg, or lifting or straining in a twisted position. Therefore, sacroiliac problems are common in running, basketball, softball, and soccer. The exaggerated pelvic rotation that some women use when working out on a stair climbing machine has also been implicated in some cases.

HISTORY AND PHYSICAL EXAMINATION

The patient presents with low back pain in the region of one or both sacroiliac joints, with or without radiation into buttocks, thigh, or groin. In the case of the patient with spondyloarthropathy, there may also be a history of monoarticular arthritis, bowel disease, iritis, or urethritis. There may be a family history of psoriasis or of spondylitis. The key physical finding in patients with sacroiliac irritation/inflammation is pain produced by stressing the sacroiliac joints either by Patrick's test, Gillet's test, or by bilateral anterior pelvic compression.[49] Patrick's test stresses the sacroiliac joint by placing the hip in flexion, abduction, and external rotation. Gillet's test is performed by placing one thumb on the S2 spinous process and the other on the posterior superior iliac spine (PSIS) on the side of suspected involvement. When flexing the hip, the normal patient's PSIS moves inferiorly to the sacral spinous process, while an abnormal sacroiliac joint will remain fixed or even elevate relative to the sacral spinous process. This maneuver may also produce pain. Muscle spasm may be present but is a nonspecific finding. In runners, the physician should measure true leg lengths. Neurologic tests will be negative, and forward and backward bending will not be painful.

ADDITIONAL STUDIES

Usually radiographs are not initially necessary if the clinical diagnosis is clear. However, when sacroiliitis is suspected but Patrick's test is negative, the physician can obtain radiographs of the sacroiliac joints. These joints are seen best on a tilted anteroposterior view of the pelvis. Tilting the pelvis anteriorly 30° puts the sacroiliac joints in the plane of the x-ray beam and allows the physician to see directly into the joints without overlap of the anterior aspect of the joint on the posterior aspect of the joint. Early inflammation will appear as osteopenia in the subchondral bone or as irregularity of the edges of the joint. Well-established sacroiliitis may reveal sclerosis and loss of joint space. Patients with long-standing sacroiliitis may have fusion of one or both sacroiliac joints. A high percentage of older, asymptomatic people show degenerative changes on plain radiographs. Bone scans can help confirm inflammation, and CT and MRI can be useful in diagnosing fracture or neoplasm, when these are suspected.

TREATMENT

Patients who have inflammatory sacroiliitis usually respond well to nonsteroidal anti-inflammatory drugs, in particular indomethacin. This can be prescribed for 2 to 3 weeks and then stopped if pain relief has been obtained. Recurrences can be treated in similar fashion. Indomethacin can be problematic in women, who may suffer from fluid retention on this drug. Nevertheless, it is very effective in treating the inflammation and should be tried. In patients with mechanical sacroiliac pain, the physician should try to determine and correct the cause. Leg-length discrepancy should be corrected within one fourth of an inch using heel and sole lifts in the running shoes. When muscle imbalance has produced a pelvic obliquity, pelvic stabilization exercises are advised to stretch the contracted side of the trunk and to strengthen the elongated side of the trunk. For the rare patient who does not respond to these measures, relief may be obtained by injection of local anesthetic and corticosteroid into the sacroiliac joint under fluoroscopic or CT guidance.[51]

FRACTURE

In the masters female athlete presenting with thoracic back pain, the physician must consider the diagnosis of pathologic or stress fractures in both ribs and vertebrae. Rib stress fractures are most common in golfers and rowers because of the repeated pull of the serratus anterior on the rib cage.[52] These fractures can occur in younger female athletes as well, but the onset of osteoporosis increases the likelihood of stress fracture. The physician must beware of attributing the stress fracture to the sport; metastatic breast cancer can also occur in both vertebrae and ribs and produce pathologic fractures.

The history and physical examination are described in the chapter on stress fractures. In addition, the physician should question the patient about previous or present breast masses or gynecologic problems and about a personal or family history of cancer.

In a woman who is middle aged or older, if no fracture is seen on plain radiograph, a complete bone scan is recommended not only to diagnose the fracture, but also to rule out other lesions. Even when the bone scan is positive only in a single rib or vertebra, the physician must consider the possibility of a metastatic lesion. If the index of suspicion is high, because of personal or family history, the patient should be referred to her primary care physician for further workup. If no underlying neoplastic process is found, the stress fracture can be treated symptomatically.

SCIATICA

Although sciatica resulting from disk herniation occurs in the female athlete, disk herniation is more common in men than in women. Furthermore, its presentation, evaluation, and treatment are no different in the female athlete than in the male athlete and will not be discussed here. On the other hand, sciatica can be a manifestation of pelvic floor dysfunction, a problem seen almost exclusively in women.

Pelvic floor dysfunction usually presents as urinary incontinence, but can also produce pain that mimics sciatica. The pelvic floor muscles include the levator ani group (pubococcygeus, puborectalis, pubovaginalis, and iliococcygeus) and the coccygeus. In addition, the piriformis and obturator internus muscles are continuous with the pelvic diaphragm made up of the above mentioned muscles. The endopelvic fascial floor and the smooth muscle diaphragm in the base of the broad ligament also contribute to the support of the pelvic floor.

There are four types of pelvic floor dysfunction: disuse, supportive, hypertonic, and incoordination.[53] Disuse dysfunction implies lack of awareness of these muscles from lack of training, modesty, or muscle imbalance; it presents as stress incontinence or urge incontinence. Supportive dysfunction is secondary to loss of nerve (pudendal), muscle, ligament, or fascial integrity. It is most commonly caused by trauma from childbirth or surgery, but can also be congenital, hormonal, or secondary to connective tissue disease. Supportive dysfunction presents as back pain and a sensation of suprapubic pressure. Hypertonic dysfunction is defined as excessive tone in the pelvic floor muscles. It can be musculoskeletal, psychogenic, or iatrogenic in origin. The primary symptom is pain that is poorly localized in the perivaginal, perirectal, or suprapubic regions and can radiate down the posterior thigh, thus making it easily confused with sciatica. Symptoms may be reproduced by a vaginal or rectal examination. Associated sexual dysfunction and dyspareunia are common. Incoordination dysfunction is difficulty in the contraction or relaxation of the pelvic floor muscles. Muscle imbalances of the gluteals, adductors, and abdominals can mask weak contraction of the pelvic floor muscles. Myofascial or scar tissue formation can restrict the contractility of the pelvic floor muscles. This can also occur from neural damage and motor dysynergia.

HISTORY AND PHYSICAL EXAMINATION

Patients present with sciatica originating from the area of the ischial tuberosity or with pain localized to the upper, outer quadrant of the buttock. The pain is not exacerbated by activities or Valsalva maneuvers. A history of urinary incontinence is common in many patients, whereas a few may experience dyspareunia. The patient is likely to be parous, and many have had traumatic vaginal deliveries.

Physical examination is more remarkable for its pertinent negative findings than positive findings. Patients with sciatica secondary to pelvic floor dysfunction have no restriction of back motion and no neurologic findings. Their hamstrings are not particularly tight and a straight leg raising test does not reproduce the sciatic pain. Occasionally, piriformis muscle tightness will be noted as manifested by decreased internal rotation of the hip on the involved side. Normally, both hips have a similar total arc of motion, although one hip may have more or less internal rotation than the other. In patients with a unilaterally tight piriformis muscle, the total arc of motion of the involved hip will be less than on the normal side, and the loss will be in internal rotation. A vaginal or rectal digital examination may reveal hypertonic or flaccid muscles. When muscles are hypertonic, the examination will be difficult to perform. When muscles are flaccid, the patient will not be able to squeeze the examining digit.

The tone of the pelvic floor muscles can be measured using perineometers or surface electromyography (EMG). These tests can also reveal whether the patient can voluntarily contract her perineal muscles in a coordinated fashion, or whether they are constantly flaccid or tonic.

TREATMENT

The initial treatment for pelvic floor dysfunction is pelvic floor muscle strengthening exercises.[54] Although many women are familiar with Kegel exercises, these exercises are often performed incorrectly.[53] Improper exercise technique causes bearing down instead of lifting up of the pelvic floor. Once the pelvic floor muscles are strengthened, the patient will be able to relax the piriformis and other gluteal muscles that have tried to take over pelvic support, but have produced sciatic compression in the process.

The principles of training the pelvic floor muscles are the same as for any other muscle—specificity, overload, and progression. Biofeedback is very useful in educating women about the use of their pelvic floor muscles. It can be supplied through use of pressure-sensing perineometers that can be inserted vaginally and that provide numeric values and visual feedback to the patient during pelvic floor muscle contractions. Surface EMG can also be used for biofeedback in the training mode.

A home program in which weighted vaginal cones are used can be instituted. Vaginal cones encourage proper lifting of the pelvic floor during contractions. These exercises are begun in positions that eliminate gravity and are advanced to upright and functional positions. They can be done concentrically, eccentrically, and isometrically and should include work on coordination as well as strengthening.[55] Women with hypertonic pelvic floor muscles benefit from biofeedback to learn how to relax these muscles.

DISSECTING AORTIC ANEURYSM

Although a dissecting aortic aneurysm is an extremely rare cause of back pain, it was just such a medical problem that led to the death of volleyball great Flo Hyman. In a patient presenting with back pain who has known Marfan syndrome or marfanoid features, the physician should always consider the possibility of aortic dissection.

At the time of this writing, bone screws placed posteriorly into vertebral elements have not been cleared for use in this specific manner by the Food and Drug Administration (FDA). These are Class III devices. This category includes screws placed transfacetally, within pedicles, or in articular, lateral masses. Some bone screws for use within the sacrum have been approved as Class II devices. Some companies have received Class II clearance for use of screws in lumbar pedicles specifically to supplement fusions in the treatment of grade III and IV spondylolisthesis with the proviso that these devices are removed after the arthrodesis has healed. Anterior vertebral body screws (cervical, thoracic, and lumbar) are Class II devices and can be used as labeled in vertebral bodies. Many of the posterior screw-based devices have been shown in laboratory and clinical testing to be useful and may be used in an off-label manner if the physician feels this is appropriate and important for the treatment of the patient. As with all surgeries, informed consent should explain the procedure and why a particular technique has been chosen, as well as its risks and benefits. The question of whether informed consent regarding pedicle screws must include a discussion of the device's FDA clearance status is currently being litigated in several jurisdictions. In cases that have been included in the multidistrict litigation in the Eastern District of Pennsylvania, this additional requirement has not been imposed.

REFERENCES

1. Micheli LJ, Wood R: Back pain in young athletes: Significant differences from adults in causes and patterns. *Arch Pediatr Adolesc Med* 1995; 149:15-18.

2. NCAA Injury Surveillance System, 1996. NCAA, 6201 College Blvd., Overland Park, KA 66211-2422.

3. Fredrickson BE, Baker D, McHolick WJ, et al: The natural history of spondylolysis and spondylolisthesis. *J Bone Joint Surg* 1984; 66A:699-707.

4. Jackson DW, Wiltse LL, Cirincione RJ: Spondylolysis in the female gymnast. *Clin Orthop* 1976;117:68-73.

5. Fehlandt AF Jr, Micheli LJ: Lumbar facet stress fracture in a ballet dancer. *Spine* 1993; 18:2537-2539.

6. Taillard WF: Etiology of spondylolisthesis. *Clin Orthop* 1976;117:30-39.

7. Kadel NJ, Teitz CC, Kronmal RA: Stress fractures in ballet dancers. *Am J Sports Med* 1992; 20:445-449.

8. Phalen GS, Dickson JA: Spondylolisthesis and tight hamstrings. *J Bone Joint Surg* 1961; 43A:505-512.

9. Bradford DS, Hu SS: Spondylolisthesis and spondylolysis, in Weinstein SL (ed): *The Pediatric Spine: Principles and Practice.* New York, NY, Raven Press, 1994, vol 1, pp 585-601.

10. Teplick JG, Laffey PA, Berman A, et al: Diagnosis and evaluation of spondylolisthesis and/or spondylolysis on axial CT. *Am J Neuroradiol* 1986;7:479-491.

11. van den Oever M, Merrick MV, Scott JH: Bone scintigraphy in symptomatic spondylolysis. *J Bone Joint Surg* 1987;69B:453-456.

12. Lowe J, Schachner E, Hirschberg E, et al: Significance of bone scintigraphy in symptomatic spondylolysis. *Spine* 1984;9:653-655.

13. Bellah RD, Summerville DA, Treves ST, et al: Low-back pain in adolescent athletes: Detection of stress injury to the pars interarticularis with SPECT. *Radiology* 1991;180:509-512.

14. Boxall D, Bradford DS, Winter RB, et al: Management of severe spondylolisthesis in children and adolescents. *J Bone Joint Surg* 1979;61A:479-495.

15. Pizzutillo PD, Hummer CD III: Nonoperative treatment for painful adolescent spondylolysis or spondylolisthesis. *J Pediatr Orthop* 1989; 9:538-540.

16. Steiner ME, Micheli LJ: Treatment of symptomatic spondylolysis and spondylolisthesis with the modified Boston brace. *Spine* 1985; 10:937-943.

17. Seitsalo S, Osterman D, Hynarinen H, et al: Progression of spondylolisthesis in children and adolescents: A long-term follow-up of 272 patients. *Spine* 1991;16:417-421.

18. Soren A, Waugh TR: Spondylolisthesis and related disorders: A correlative study of 105 patients. *Clin Orthop* 1985;193:171-177.

19. Ciullo JV, Jackson DW: Pars interarticularis stress reaction, spondylolysis, and spondylolisthesis in gymnasts. *Clin Sports Med* 1985; 4:95-110.

20. Wiltse LL: Spondylolisthesis: Classification and etiology, in American Academy of Orthopaedic Surgeons (ed): *Symposium on the Spine.* St. Louis, MO, CV Mosby, 1969, pp 143-167.

21. Iknoian T: Pilates technique. *Women's Sports and Fitness* 1992;14:63.

22. Pizzutillo PD, Mirenda W, MacEwen GD: Posterolateral fusion for spondylolisthesis in adolescence. *J Pediatr Orthop* 1986;6:311-316.

23. Frennered AK, Danielson BI, Nachemson AL, et al: Midterm follow-up of young patients fused in situ for spondylolisthesis. *Spine* 1991; 16:409-416.

24. Burkus JK, Lonstein JE, Winter RB, et al: Long-term evaluation of adolescents treated operatively for spondylolisthesis: A comparison of in situ arthrodesis only with in situ arthrodesis and reduction followed by immobilization in a cast. *J Bone Joint Surg* 1992;74A:693-704.

25. Bradford DS, Gotfried Y: Staged salvage reconstruction of grade IV and V spondylolisthesis. *J Bone Joint Surg* 1987;69A:191-202.

26. Pedersen AK, Hagen R: Spondylolysis and spondylolisthesis: Treatment by internal fixation and bone-grafting of the defect. *J Bone Joint Surg* 1988;70A:15-24.

27. Winter M, Jani L: Results of screw osteosynthesis in spondylolysis and low-grade spondylolisthesis. *Arch Orthop Trauma Surg* 1989; 108:96-99.

28. Johnson GV, Thompson AG: The Scott wiring technique for direct repair of lumbar spondylolysis. *J Bone Joint Surg* 1992;74B:426-430.

29. Hensinger RN, Lang JR, MacEwen GD: Surgical management of spondylolisthesis in children and adolescents. *Spine* 1976;1:207-216.

30. Asher M, Green P, Orrick J: A six-year report: Spinal deformity screening in Kansas school children. *J Kans Med Soc* 1980;81:568-571.

31. Lonstein JE, Bjorklund S, Wanninger MH, et al: Voluntary school screening for scoliosis in Minnesota. *J Bone Joint Surg* 1982;64A:481-488.

32. Warren MP, Brooks-Gunn J, Hamilton LH, et al: Scoliosis and fractures in young ballet dancers: Relation to delayed menarche and secondary amenorrhea. *N Engl J Med* 1986;314:1348-1353.

33. MacEwen GD, Cowell HR: Familial incidence of idiopathic scoliosis and its implications in patient treatment. *J Bone Joint Surg* 1970; 52A:405.

34. Collis DK, Ponseti IV: Long-term follow-up of patients with idiopathic scoliosis not treated surgically. *J Bone Joint Surg* 1969;51A:425-445.

35. Nachemson AL, Peterson LE: Effectiveness of treatment with a brace in girls who have adolescent idiopathic scoliosis: A prospective, controlled study based on data from the Brace Study of the Scoliosis Research Society. *J Bone Joint Surg* 1995;77A:815-822.

36. Cochran T, Irstam L, Nachemson A: Long-term anatomic and functional changes in patients with adolescent idiopathic scoliosis treated by Harrington rod fusion. *Spine* 1983;8:576-584.

37. Lenke LG, Bridwell KH, Baldus C, et al: Preventing decompensation in King type II curves treated with Cotrel-Dubousset instrumentation: Strict guidelines for selective thoracic fusion. *Spine* 1992;17(suppl 8):S274-S281.

38. Richards BS, Birch JG, Herring JA, et al: Frontal plane and sagittal plane balance following Cotrel-Dubousset instrumentation for idiopathic scoliosis. *Spine* 1989;14:733-737.

39. Dwyer AF, Newton NC, Sherwood AA: An anterior approach to scoliosis: A preliminary report. *Clin Orthop* 1969;62:192-202.

40. Kaneda K, Fujiya N, Satoh S: Results with Zielke instrumentation for idiopathic thoracolumbar and lumbar scoliosis. *Clin Orthop* 1986; 205:195-203.

41. Moe JH, Purcell GA, Bradford DS: Zielke instrumentation (VDS) for the correction of spinal curvature: Analysis of results in 66 patients. *Clin Orthop* 1983;180:133-153.

42. Lagrone MO, Bradford DS, Moe JH, et al: Treatment of symptomatic flatback after spinal fusion. *J Bone Joint Surg* 1988;70A:569-580.

43. Micheli LJ: Low back pain in the adolescent: Differential diagnosis. *Am J Sports Med* 1979; 7:362-364.

44. Teitz CC, Cook DM: Rehabilitation of neck and low back injuries. *Clin Sports Med* 1985; 4:455-476.

45. McKenzie RA: Prophylaxis in recurrent low back pain. *NZ Med J* 1979;89:22-23.

46. Donelson R: The McKenzie approach to evaluating and treating low back pain. *Orthop Rev* 1990;19:681-686.

47. Bernard TN, Cassidy JD: The sacroiliac joint syndrome: Pathophysiology, diagnosis, and management, in Frymoyer JW (ed): *The Adult Spine: Principles and Practice.* New York, NY, Raven Press,1991, pp 2107-2130.

48. Schumacher HR Jr (ed): *Primer on the Rheumatic Diseases,* ed 9. Atlanta, GA, Arthritis Foundation, 1988, pp 142-155.

49. Colliton J: Back pain and pregnancy: Active management strategies. *Phys Sportsmed* 1996; 24:89-93.

50. Fortin JD, Aprill CN, Ponthieux RT, et al: Sacroiliac joint: Pain referral maps upon applying a new injection/arthrography technique. Part II: Clinical evaluation. *Spine* 1994; 19:1483-1489.

51. Bernard TN, Kirkaldy-Willis WH: Recognizing specific characteristics of nonspecific low back pain. *Clin Orthop* 1987;217:266-280.

52. Holden DL, Jackson DW: Stress fractures of the ribs in female rowers. *Am J Sports Med* 1985;13:342-348.

53. Wallace K: Female pelvic floor functions, dysfunctions, and behavioral approaches to treatment. *Clin Sports Med* 1994;13:459-481.

54. Kegel AH: Progressive resistance exercise in the functional restoration of the perineal muscles. *Am J Obstet Gynecol* 1948;56:238-248.

55. Nygaard I: Prevention of exercise incontinence with mechanical devices. *J Reprod Med* 1995;40:89-94.

THE UPPER EXTREMITIES

CAROL C. TEITZ, MD

THE SHOULDER

Two problems in the shoulder present more commonly in the female athlete. One is impingement in swimmers; the other is thoracic outlet syndrome in athletes with long thin necks, especially dancers.[1,2]

IMPINGEMENT

Shoulder pain secondary to impingement is more common in female than in male swimmers, especially those swimming crawl and butterfly.[3] Two hypothetical sources for an increased potential for subacromial impingement include increased ligamentous laxity and relative body size. Women with increased flexibility are at risk for subacromial impingement as a result of increased glenohumeral motion. Furthermore, because of her relatively shorter body length, the female swimmer requires more strokes than her male counterpart to cover the same distance in the pool. The need for more strokes obviously increases the exposure of the subacromial tissues to the potential for impingement.

The presentation, diagnosis, and treatment of impingement are no different in the female athlete than in the male. However, the physician should consider the possibility of increased glenohumeral motion as an etiologic factor in women. The increased laxity noted above may also account for voluntary shoulder dislocation occurring more commonly in females. Therefore, when treating overt instability or symptoms of impingement caused by instability, the orthopaedist should try shoulder girdle strengthening exercises for quite a while before considering any surgical procedure to increase the subacromial space or stabilize the glenohumeral joint. A soft-tissue stabilization procedure is more likely to stretch out in the female athlete than in the male (see "The Knee" for tests for generalized laxity).

THORACIC OUTLET SYNDROME

Shoulder pain can also be caused by thoracic outlet syndrome (TOS), which is three times more common in women than in men.[4] The thoracic outlet extends from the supraclavicular fossa to the axilla and includes the space between the clavicle and the first rib bounded by the anterior scalene muscle and the apex of the lung. Through this outlet pass the subclavian artery and vein and the brachial plexus. Any condition that causes poor suspension of the shoulder girdle, a relatively depressed scapula, and tension on the scalene muscles can produce compression of the neurovascular structures exiting the thoracic outlet. In women, this may be caused by a long asthenic neck, relatively weak shoulder girdle musculature, or excessively large breasts.[5] A weak trapezius muscle can result from a neck injury.[6] Moreover, any injury that causes the patient to guard the upper extremity can produce disuse atrophy of supporting shoulder girdle muscles. Less commonly, compression of the neurovascular structures in the thoracic outlet is caused by an embryologic fibrotic band between a spinous process and the clavicle, anomalous insertions of the scalenes into the clavicle, or by a cervical rib.

History and Physical Examination

The symptoms of TOS depend on the structure(s) entrapped. These symptoms may range from neck and shoulder pain to arm pain and numbness. Hand weakness may occur, especially when the arm is held in an abducted position. Sometimes, circulatory changes are noted, but are not necessary to make the diagnosis. Nocturnal pain is common and can make the physician think of carpal tunnel syndrome. The "dead arm syndrome" secondary to glenohumeral instability may produce symptoms similar to those of TOS.[7]

On physical examination the physician should first look to see if the clavicles appear relatively horizontal (a sign of a depressed scapula) rather than elevating at their acromial ends. In some patients, the ipsilateral scapula will be obviously lower than on the asymptomatic side. Many patients have a long neck with a "forward head."

The physician should check the vascular supply to the limb as well as performing a careful neurologic examination. Most commonly, TOS involves the lower trunk of the brachial plexus and may produce decreased sensation in the distribution of the medial brachial or medial antebrachial cutaneous nerves. Finding decreased sensation in the areas supplied by these nerves helps to differentiate the problem from an ulnar neuropathy. Similarly, carpal tunnel syndrome would produce symptoms and signs on the radial side of the hand rather than on the ulnar side. The latter are more common in patients with TOS. C8 radiculopathy would be manifest by weakness of the thenar muscles supplied by the recurrent branch of the median nerve in addition to weakness of the intrinsics supplied by the ulnar nerve.

A series of provocative abduction tests (Adson's test, Wright's test) have been described for both the subclavian artery and the brachial plexus (Fig. 21). Wright's test should also be done with the elbow straight so as not to produce symptoms related to the ulnar nerve stretching around a flexed elbow. Bracing the shoulder in a military position or pressing down on the shoulder may reproduce symptoms in patients with decreased space between the clavicle and the first rib. When any of the stress maneuvers reproduce the patient's symptoms, TOS is likely.

Additional Studies

Anteroposterior (AP) and lateral radiographs of the neck should be taken. On the lateral view, the physician should note the presence of disk space narrowing. Radiographs of the neck taken without any downward traction on the arms will often reveal all seven cervical vertebrae and even T1 in some patients. This is diagnostic of "droopy shoulders." The additional finding of horizontal clavicles on the AP radiograph supports the diagnosis of a depressed scapula. When the apices of the lung are not visible on the AP radiograph of the neck, an additional AP radiograph of the chest or an apical lordotic radiograph of the chest should be taken to rule out compression from an apical lung tumor, such as Pancoast's tumor. Nerve conduction velocity tests are not typically helpful, but may reveal a nerve root impingement

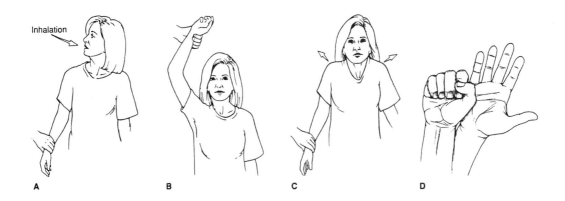

FIGURE 21

Provocative maneuvers used in evaluation of patients with suspected TOS. Symptoms must be reproduced for tests to be considered positive. **A,** Adson's maneuver. **B,** Wright's maneuver. **C,** Costoclavicular, or military brace, maneuver. **D,** Overhead exercise test. (Reproduced with permission from Leffert RD: Thoracic outlet syndrome. *J Am Acad Orthop Surg* 1994;2:317-325.)

rather than TOS. Magnetic resonance imaging, computed tomography, and somatosensory evoked potentials are rarely useful in diagnosis.[8] Vascular studies are necessary only when there is strong evidence of vascular pathology.

Treatment

Initial treatment should be directed at elevating the shoulder girdle and decreasing the tension on the scalene muscles.[9] Strengthening exercises should be prescribed for the trapezius, rhomboids, and levator scapulae. Care must be taken not to prescribe exercises with the arm overhead. Learning to retract the head posteriorly with erector spinae muscles is also helpful in establishing a more physiologic relationship between the neck and the shoulder. Patients need to be encouraged because symptoms may not change for 2 months after beginning an appropriate exercise program. Women with large breasts should consider wearing longline bras, which support the weight of the breasts from below rather than from the shoulder, or undergoing reduction mammoplasty.

In patients who fail to respond to nonsurgical therapy, or in those with significant neurologic deficits or serious vascular signs, surgical treatment is recommended.[10] Scalenotomy or scalenectomy with first rib resection has met with success in 82% of patients who failed nonsurgical treatment.[10] Patients who are found to have an accessory rib or fibrotic band should have it removed.

THE WRIST

Chronic wrist pain is common in the gymnast and is thought to result from using the upper extremity to bear weight. In college-age gymnasts, wrist problems are more prevalent in males and include ligamentous tears in the triangular fibrocartilage complex, chondromalacia of the ulnarlunate, ulnar-triquetral, and radio-scaphoid articulations.[11,12] In younger adolescent gymnasts, wrist pain is more prevalent in females[13] and is more often found to be caused by stress fractures of the distal radial physis.[14] This problem was initially described by Roy and associates[15] who identified changes in the distal radial physis of the skeletally immature gymnast. Subsequent studies have revealed positive ulnar variance in these gym-

nasts, which is thought to be caused by premature closure of the radial physis.[16]

Although the cause of the increased prevalence of physeal injuries in girls is unknown, DiFiori and associates[13] found that the girls with this problem started training at a later age and trained more hours per week than the boys in their study. Starting training at an "older" age (eg, 9 years) places girls who are about to enter their growth spurt in a situation of trying to catch up with their chronologic peers and perhaps spending more time practicing upper extremity support and wrist impacting activities. Sixty-six percent of DiFiori and associates'[13] subjects with wrist pain were between the ages of 10 and 14 years, and more than 93% of gymnasts in this age range had wrist pain.

HISTORY AND PHYSICAL EXAMINATION

The gymnast presents with wrist pain, which is made worse by activity that involves bearing weight on the upper extremities, especially in extremes of dorsiflexion, such as tumbling. Vaults and balance beam routines that involve rotation as well as dorsiflexion are particularly problematic.

Physical examination reveals decreased dorsiflexion and sometimes pain on forced volarflexion as well. Swelling is typically absent but tenderness will be localized over the distal radial epiphysis rather than over the carpal bones or triangular fibrocartilage. There typically is no evidence of ganglions, tendinitis, or abnormal laxity of the radioulnar joint.

ADDITIONAL TESTS

Radiographs reveal widening of the distal radial physis, particularly radially and volarly. Cysts may be seen on the metaphyseal side of the physis and beaking on the epiphyseal side. Occasionally, haziness is noted in what is usually a lucent area in the physis. These changes are thought to represent stress fracture of the distal radial physis (Fig. 22).[16] Radiographs in the skeletally mature gymnast with chronic wrist pain may reveal a relatively long ulna.[17-19]

TREATMENT

When the patient is seen early and has clinical signs, but normal radiographs, abstaining from weightbearing on the upper extremities usually results in cessation of symptoms in about 3 to 4 weeks. Once radiographic changes are noted,

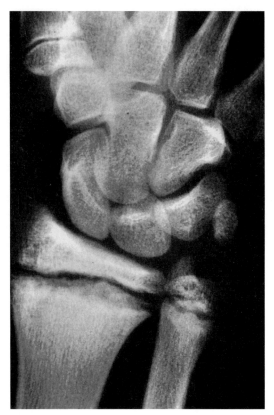

FIGURE 22

An anteroposterior radiograph reveals cyst formation and widening of the distal radial physis.

it may take 3 to 6 months of nonweightbearing to become asymptomatic. Splinting or casting is needed only rarely. The gymnast can continue to work out doing aerials on floor and beam, but needs to stay off vault and tumbling. She should refrain from bearing weight on the involved upper extremity until her wrist is nontender and is not painful during forced dorsiflexion. Once the gymnast returns to activity, her wrist should be taped to prevent forced dorsiflexion. Initially, dorsiflexion maneuvers such as handstands and walkovers should be done in limited number. Vaulting should be avoided for about 3 weeks after return to activity. Twisting vaults and twisting maneuvers on beam should be avoided for a longer period of time.

REFERENCES

1. Schulte KR, Warner JJ: Uncommon causes of shoulder pain in the athlete. *Orthop Clin North Am* 1995;26:505-528.

2. Hoppmann RA, Reid RR: Musculoskeletal problems of performing artists. *Curr Opin Rheumatol* 1995;7:147-150.

3. Kennedy JC, Hawkins R, Krissoff WB: Orthopaedic manifestations of swimming. *Am J Sports Med* 1978;6:309-322.

4. Leffert RD: Thoracic outlet syndrome. *J Am Acad Orthop Surg* 1994;2:317-325.

5. Kaye BL: Neurologic changes with excessively large breasts. *South Med J* 1972;65:177-180.

6. Magnusson T: Extracervical symptoms after whiplash trauma. *Cephalalgia* 1994;14:223-227.

7. Leffert RD, Gumley G: The relationship between dead arm syndrome and thoracic outlet syndrome. *Clin Orthop* 1987;223:20-31.

8. Veilleux M, Stevens JC, Campbell JK: Somatosensory evoked potentials: Lack of value for diagnosis of thoracic outlet syndrome. *Muscle Nerve* 1988;11:571-575.

9. Liebenson CS: Thoracic outlet syndrome: Diagnosis and conservative management. *J Manipulative Physiol Ther* 1988;11:493-499.

10. Cina C, Whiteacre L, Edwards R, et al: Treatment of thoracic outlet syndrome with combined scalenectomy and transaxillary first-rib resection. *Cardiovasc Surg* 1994;2:514-518.

11. Mandelbaum BR, Bartolozzi AR, Davis CA, et al: Wrist pain syndrome in the gymnast: Pathogenetic, diagnostic, and therapeutic considerations. *Am J Sports Med* 1989;17:305-317.

12. Weiker GG: Hand and wrist problems in the gymnast. *Clin Sports Med* 1992;11:189-202.

13. DiFiori JP, Puffer JC, Mandelbaum BR, et al: Factors associated with wrist pain in the young gymnast. *Am J Sports Med* 1996;24:9-14.

14. Caine D, Roy S, Singer KM, et al: Stress changes of the distal radial growth plate: A radiographic survey and review of the literature. *Am J Sports Med* 1992;20:290-298.

15. Roy S, Caine D, Singer KM: Stress changes of the distal radial epiphysis in young gymnasts: A report of 21 cases and a review of the literature. *Am J Sports Med* 1985;13:301-308.

16. Shih C, Chang CY, Penn IW, et al: Chronically stressed wrists in adolescent gymnasts: MR imaging appearance. *Radiology* 1995; 195:855-859.

17. Tolat AR, Sanderson PL, DeSmet L, et al: The gymnast's wrist: Acquired positive ulnar variance following chronic epiphyseal injury. *J Hand Surg* 1992;17B:678-681.

18. De Smet L, Claessens A, Lefevre J, et al: Gymnasts wrist: An epidemiologic survey of ulnar variance and stress changes of the radial physis in elite female gymnasts. *Am J Sports Med* 1994;22:846-850.

19. Chang CY, Shih C, Penn IW, et al: Wrist injuries in adolescent gymnasts of a Chinese opera school: Radiographic survey. *Radiology* 1995;195:861-864.

THE LOWER EXTREMITIES

ELIZABETH A. ARENDT, MD AND CAROL C. TEITZ, MD

THE KNEE

Common knee problems in the female athlete include patellofemoral pain, patellar subluxation and dislocation, and anterior cruciate ligament injury. Patellar problems are more common in sports involving running, although dancers, cyclists, and some swimmers (breaststrokers) also suffer from patellar problems. The masters female athlete is more likely to have pain related to osteoarthritis.

PATELLOFEMORAL PAIN

Patellofemoral pain is a global term used to describe anterior knee pain that originates in the extensor mechanism, including the patella, femur, quadriceps, and patellar retinacula.[1] The increased prevalence in women is attributed to the difference in lower-extremity alignment between the average man and the average woman.[2,3] In addition to inherited variations, such as the degree of femoral anteversion or genu valgum, changes in the breadth of the pelvis occur in the female during puberty (and later during pregnancy). The period during which these changes take place in girls is shorter than the growth period in adolescent boys.[4,5] This period of accelerated body changes can produce changes in sport performance as girls accommodate to their new shapes. While the hips broaden in females, the shoulders broaden in pubertal males. Interestingly, elite, successful female and male track and field athletes have been found to have similar physiques in regard to relative hip and shoulder width.[6]

Although pelvic size and width vary widely within each sex as well as between the sexes, in general, women have wider dimensions of the true pelvis to accommodate childbirth. Because of the broader pelvis in women, the lower extremities assume a more valgus position at the knee, with subsequent pronation at the foot. In addition, in females there is a higher prevalence of increased femoral anteversion which, in turn,

affects the biomechanics of the patellofemoral joint (Fig. 23).[7] Increased femoral anteversion is hereditary and is also more common in firstborns and children who presented in a breech position at the time of birth.[8] Increased femoral anteversion and a "wide" pelvis are associated with an increased quadriceps angle (Q angle).[9] This angle, defined as the number of degrees between a line down the center of the thigh, and a line down the center of the patellar tendon is

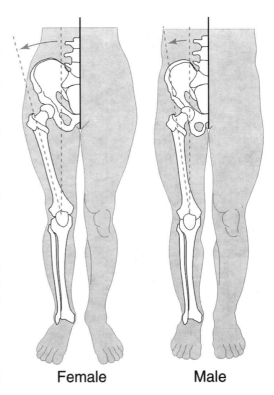

Female   Male

FIGURE 23
Females have a higher prevalence of increased pelvic width, femoral anteversion, and an increased Q-angle.

usually 10° in males and 15° in females. The Q angle determines in part the tracking of the patella in the femoral trochlea. Tracking is also determined in part by the relative balance of the vastus medialis obliquus and the vastus lateralis, the depth of the trochlear groove, and the tightness of the retinaculum, including attachments of the iliotibial band to the lateral side of the patella.[10-12] When excessive femoral anteversion is present, there is often compensatory increased external tibial torsion and subsequent pronation in order to achieve a plantigrade position of the foot. This triad is termed "miserable malalignment"[13] (Fig. 24). Because of the way the foot contacts the ground, ie, pronating too early, there is increased rotation of the tibia during running. Some authors believe that this increased rotation of the tibia leads to increased patellar motion (resulting from the attachment of the patellar tendon to the tibial tubercle) and subsequent patellar "irritation."[13]

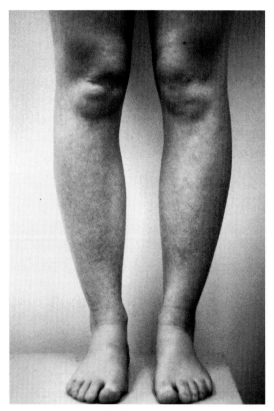

FIGURE 24
Miserable malalignment includes excessive femoral anteversion, external tibial torsion, and a pronated foot.

Another reason for patellofemoral pain is excessive lateral patellar tilt and subsequent "lateral patellar compression," which can lead to a syndrome of pain thought to represent overload of the bone in the lateral patellar facet.[14,15]

History and Physical Examination

Athletes with patellofemoral problems present with diffuse anterior knee pain, which typically is aggravated by their sport or by sitting for long periods of time with the knees flexed (positive theatre sign). There usually is no specific injury history, although there may be a history of recent increase or change in activity. A positive family history may also be forthcoming.

In addition to the usual components of a knee examination, the physician should pay particular attention to lower extremity alignment, patellar mobility, and generalized ligamentous laxity. With the patient in the standing position, the examiner should look for "cross-eyed" or "wall-eyed" patellae, a reflection of anteverted or retroverted hips, respectively. The feet should be assessed for increased hindfoot valgus or midfoot pronation.

On examination of the prone patient, the physician can assess femoral version and tibial torsion.[7] Increased internal rotation relative to external rotation of the hips reflects increased femoral anteversion. A thigh–foot angle greater than + 10° implies excessive external tibial torsion. Particularly in the adolescent, the physician should also look at the tightness of the rectus femoris using Ely's test (Fig. 25).[16] Ober's test (Fig. 26) should be performed with the patient lying on her side to assess tightness of the iliotibial bands.[17]

The physician should assess patellar retinacular tightness, which can affect patellar translation as well as patellar tilt, in the supine patient. Normal translation allows the examiner to move the patella medially about one quarter the diameter of the patella, and laterally about one half the diameter of the patella. On the other hand, when the lateral restraints (vastus lateralis, iliotibial band, and retinaculum) are tight, decreased medial translation may occur in addition to patellar tilt. When more than a fourth of the medial patellar surface is readily palpable, the patella usually is tilted downward on its lateral side. Similarly, when the lateral border of the patella cannot be placed in the horizontal plane or angled upward

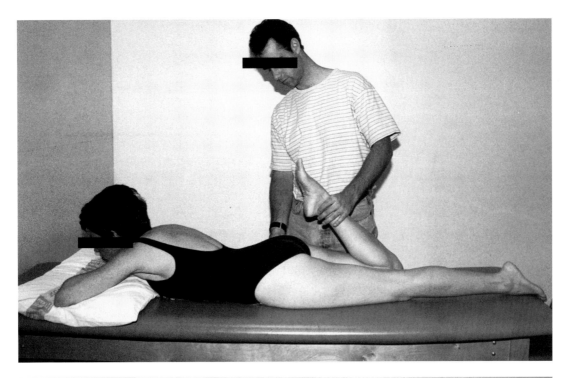

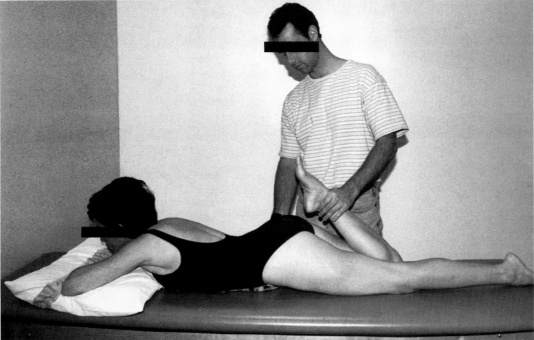

FIGURE 25

Ely's test. When the rectus femoris is tight, attempts to bring the heel to the buttock will result in anterior tilt of the pelvis. **Top,** Normal. **Bottom,** Positive Ely's test.

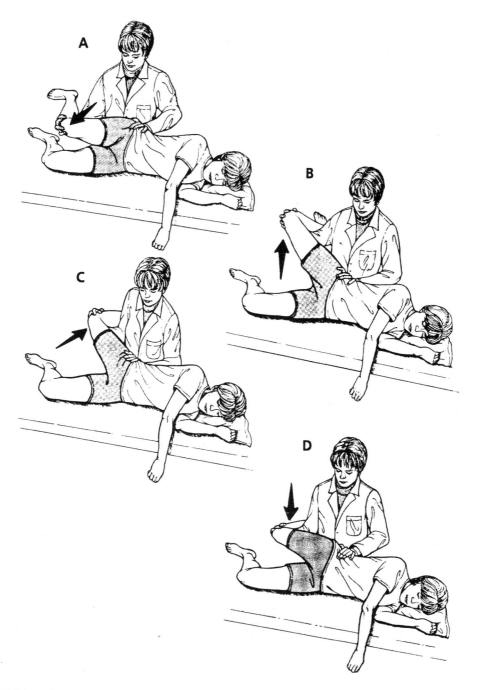

FIGURE 26

Ober's test. In Ober's test, the patient lies on the unaffected side with the unaffected hip and knee flexed to eliminate lumbar lordosis. The examiner holds the leg with the knee flexed, while the other hand stabilizes the patient's pelvis. The leg is flexed (**A**), abducted (**B**), and hyperextended (**C**) to catch the iliotibial band on the greater trochanter, then adducted (**D**). If the iliotibial band is tight, the leg cannot be adducted back down to the table or opposite leg. (Reproduced with permission from Teitz CC: Diagnosing and managing common dance injuries. *J Musculoskel Med* 1996;13:46-57.)

on its lateral side 15°, the lateral retinaculum is tight.[15] The examiner should attempt to locate sites of tenderness (patellar facets, trochlea, retinaculum, plicae). The Q angle can be measured in the extended knee position, but should be measured again with the knee at 30° of flexion, where the patella should engage the trochlea. Swelling may be present. Hamstring tightness should be assessed using a straight leg raising test. Hamstring tightness is a common finding in the adolescent in the midst of a growth spurt. In the sitting patient, the physician should remeasure the Q angle and palpate the knee for crepitus during range of motion. Crepitus that feels "fine" like granola or crinkling tissue paper and is palpable through the entire arc of knee motion is associated with synovitis, ie, inflammation. On the other hand, coarse clicks and pops are common and have no association with any specific physical finding unless the patella is felt to "jump" at a reproducible, specific point in the range of motion. When this occurs between 30° and 60°, there may a surface irregularity on the patella or trochlea or a horizontal plica may be present, but their clinical significance is debatable.[1]

The patient should be watched while extending her knee from 90° to full extension. The patella should stay centrally located throughout the range with a slight lateral jog in the last 5° to 10° of extension caused by the screw home mechanism of the knee. When the patella moves medially or when lateral movement occurs earlier, there usually is a muscular imbalance, tight lateral retinacular restraints, or significant bony abnormalities, including a relatively flat trochlea. These may make patellar subluxation and dislocation more likely.[18,19]

Generalized ligamentous laxity can be estimated by looking for the following five signs: ability to hyperflex the thumb against the ipsilateral forearm, hyperextension of the fifth metacarpophalangeal joint beyond 90°, recurvatum of the elbows and knees, and flat feet. The patient who has three or more of these findings has generalized laxity.[20] Patients with patellofemoral pain and radiographic malalignment should be differentiated from those without radiographic malalignment.

Additional Studies

Radiographic examination should include anteroposterior (AP), lateral, and axial views of the knee. On the lateral view, the physician should look for patella alta (Insall's ratio) and any irregularities in the patellofemoral surfaces. The axial views can demonstrate patellar subluxation[21] and suggest patellar tilt when the medial facet is elevated away from the medial trochlea.[1] They may also demonstrate increased density in the lateral patellar facet, which is thought to represent increased compression of the subchondral bone laterally. This increased density is often associated with lateral patellar tilt.[15] Recently, computed tomography and magnetic resonance imaging (MRI) have made it possible to view the patella during earlier phases of knee flexion than was possible with traditional radiographs, and to control the limb for anteversion.[18,22-24] However, a large amount of variability remains in and between these studies, indicating a need for further research in this area.

Treatment

The key to treatment of patellofemoral pain seems to be balancing the movement of the patella so that it tracks centrally in the trochlear groove.[25,26] Quadriceps strengthening is a long-standing and well-accepted method for treating patellofemoral pain.[27] However, a common error that is made in prescribing quadriceps exercises is the use of isotonic exercises early in the rehabilitation phase when these exercises may aggravate patellofemoral pain.[28] Initial emphasis should be placed on isometric exercise, advancing to closed kinetic chain isotonic exercise. Closed kinetic chain exercises more closely simulate the tibial rotation and subtalar motion that occur during functional activities.[29,30] In addition, lower patellar contact stresses have been demonstrated in mid-arc closed chain exercises than in open chain exercises.[31]

Electrical stimulation can be used for patients who cannot initiate a good quadriceps contraction.[32] McConnell taping also may assist patients who have pain while trying to do quadriceps-strengthening exercises. Developed by an Australian physical therapist, this type of taping is based on an assessment and tape correction of patellar position and tracking in glide, tilt, and rotation.[33] The use of patellar braces in these patients remains controversial.[28,34] Because the vastus lateralis often is stronger than the vastus medialis, and because the vastus medialis obliquus is known to fire during the last 30° of knee extension,[35] short arc isotonic exercises are also emphasized. During sports, the quadriceps frequently contracts eccentrically, particularly where deceleration is required (the jumping athlete). In one study, less patellofemoral pain was reported when the ratio of eccentric to concentric quadriceps strength was one or more during isokinetic testing.[36] Therefore, eccentric training is important. However, it should be reserved until later in the rehabilitation program because patellofemoral forces are higher during eccentric training and it may increase pain when other factors have not yet been corrected. In addition to quadriceps strengthening, however, treatment should be more specific and individualized based on the findings during physical examination (Table 6). In adolescent girls with anterior knee pain, normal alignment, a dearth of physical findings, and no response to the usual treatments, the physician should consider reflex sympathetic dystrophy (see "Disproportionate Pain Syndromes" p. 90).

Surgical treatment of patellofemoral pain should be limited to those patients who demonstrate radiographic malalignment. Lateral retinacular releases have been helpful in relieving patellar tilt.[37] Excision of a symptomatic plica should be reserved for patients in whom a reproducible click always is noted at the same degree of knee flexion, and in whom nonsteroidal anti-inflammatory drugs (NSAIDs) and ice massage have provided no relief. Arthroscopic patellar shaving is indicated when effusion is present and cannot be controlled with NSAIDs. Shaving should be combined with procedures to unload stressed areas of patellar articular cartilage. The role of long-bone osteotomy in the treatment of patellar pain is still in early stages of investigation. When the radiographic relationship betweeen the patella and trochlear groove is normal, the patella is stable, and rotational malalignment is present, the physician should consider an extra-articular long bone osteotomy to decrease pain.[38]

Sport-Specific Treatment

When swimmers, particularly breaststrokers, complain of anterior knee pain, it often is related to the whip kick. Breaststrokers who create too much of a valgus position with their knees will exaggerate any tendency for lateral patellar positioning. The swimmer should be retrained to kick with the legs in a slightly more vertical position.[39]

The cyclist with anterior knee pain ideally should have a "bike fit" done. This includes an

TABLE 6

PHYSICAL EXAMINATION FINDINGS AND TREATMENTS

Finding	Treatment
Tight patellar restraints	Refer to physical therapist for patellar mobilization
Positive Ober's test	ITB* stretches
Positive Ely's test	Rectus femoris stretches
Tight hamstrings	Hamstring stretching
Tender plica	Ice-friction massage/ NSAIDs†/steroid
Effusion	NSAIDs†/arthroscopic debridement
Pronated feet	Orthotic arch supports

* ITB, iliotibial band
† NSAIDs, nonsteroidal anti-inflammatory drugs

assessment of the position of the feet on the pedals, the height of the seat, the size of the bike frame relative to the rider, and the position of the handlebars. When patellofemoral pain is present, the athlete can first try riding in lower gear so that there is less resistance. The seat should be raised such that the knee is 20° shy of full extension at the bottom of the down stroke or such that the hips don't wobble back and forth on the seat. In addition, feet should be fixed to the pedals so the rider can use her hamstring muscles. However, attention should be paid to the relative alignment of the knees over the feet. Bike shops often place the foot fixation in a slightly internally rotated position. For cyclists with retroversion, the knees will rotate lateral to the foot; for cyclists with excessive anteversion, the knees will rotate medial to the foot. Either one can be a problem and foot fixation should be adjusted so that the knees drop over the center of the foot. The foot should be allowed to rotate 6° so it can move with the tibia as it rotates with knee motion.

In dancers, patellofemoral pain typically is caused either by poor positioning of the knees and feet or by excessive use of the quadriceps femoris.[40] No matter the type of dance, most dancers do a large series of pliés (squats, both mini and full) as a warmup. Pliés are also part of all turns and jumps. Generally, lower extremity turn out (external rotation) is emphasized, particularly in ballet. Dancers whose hips do not turn out naturally may attempt to get turn out by planting the feet in the required positions, and then torquing the knees. During the pliés, a plumb line dropped from the knees will land medial to the second toe, producing a valgus force vector on the patella while also increasing strain on the medial retinacular structures. This positioning problem can be corrected by pointing out to the dancer how much external rotation she has in her hips, where her feet should be, and that her knees should always be over her feet. In addition, she can be taught how to use the short external rotators of the hip to try to increase turn out properly. When dancers are in the extension phase of plié, ie, returning from the squat to the upright position, they should be using adductors, gluteals, and some quadriceps to return to the extended knee position. Dancers who use only their quadriceps usually develop anterior knee pain. This should be looked for by feeling the dancer's thighs during pliés. If no use of the adductors is noted, the dancer should be taught to contract these muscles, either by applying gentle manual pressure between the knees as the dancer straightens her legs, or by asking her to imagine having a ball between her knees that she will squeeze as she moves upward from the plié position. Physical therapists who are familiar with dance, or certified movement analysts can help dancers repattern their muscle use. Aerobic dancers should be told to refrain from lunges, and to stay on the lowest step if they are doing step aerobics.

PATELLAR DISLOCATION AND SUBLUXATION

Patellar dislocation and subluxation can occur from a strong valgus or external rotation force or with very little force in a hyperlax individual. Although women in general have greater ligamentous laxity, there is no documentation in the literature of differences between men and women in the incidence of first patellar dislocation. Women, however, have a higher incidence of recurrent dislocation.[41,42] Whether this incidence is due to anatomic differences, treatment and activity differences, or other factors is spec-

ulative at this time. Prognosis is not totally predictable because in the literature, dislocations are not classified with regard to bony abnormalities, chondral lesions, bone bruises, and retinacular disruption.[41,43] MRI may help in future outcome studies.[44-46]

Patella alta is associated with a higher incidence of patellar subluxation[1,10] because more knee flexion occurs before the patella engages the trochlear groove. The biomechanics of the patellofemoral joint are affected by patella alta as well. The patella increases the quadriceps' leverage at the knee by increasing the distance of the quadriceps tendon from the center of motion of the knee joint (Fig. 27). In patients with patella alta, the mechanical efficiency of the quadriceps muscle is decreased, and the patellofemoral force is increased.

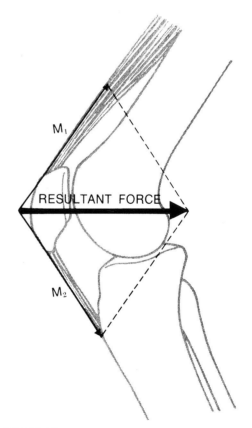

FIGURE 27
Biomechanics of the patellofemoral joint. (Reproduced with permission from Fulkerson JP, Hungerford DS (eds): *Disorders of the Patellofemoral Joint*, ed 2. Baltimore, MD, Williams & Wilkins, 1990).

History and Physical Examination

The athlete generally presents with a swollen, painful knee following some sort of noncontact rotational injury. In addition to looking for predisposing anatomic factors noted above, the physician should palpate the medial retinaculum for defects. The examiner should also attempt to move the patella laterally while holding the knee in 20° of flexion. Patients who have had a patellar subluxation or dislocation usually become apprehensive during this test. Assessing patellar tracking actively is critical, yet tracking is poorly understood. Most studies have been done in vitro and fail to take into account the dynamic action of the quadriceps muscle in vivo.

Additional Studies

The knee should be aspirated to remove the blood and to examine it for fat droplets, which may indicate a fracture even when it is not seen on radiographs. The physician should obtain radiographs, including AP, lateral, and axial views to rule out patellar fracture and to look at alignment. The AP radiograph should be taken with the patient standing unless pain limits weight-bearing. In addition to static radiographic assessment of patellofemoral congruence mentioned above, recent investigators have attempted to demonstrate dynamic patellofemoral relationships using kinematic MRI.[24] Nevertheless, good intertest reliability or a data base of asymptomatic knees to which to compare the findings in symptomatic knees currently does not exist.

Treatment

Whether all retinacular tears need surgical repair is debatable.[1,47] When loose bodies are noted, however, they should be removed using arthroscopic techniques. The surgeon can consider at that time whether lateral release, medial reef with repair of the medial patellofemoral ligament,[48] or tibial tubercle transfer is needed.[49] This decision is based on anatomic and radiographic alignment as well as on whether or not this is a recurrent dislocation. When generalized ligamentous laxity is present, the physician should remember that soft-tissue reefings are likely to stretch out as the tissues remodel with the patient's innately lax collagen. Patients with trochlear dysplasia and those with ligamentous laxity are the most difficult to treat.

Patients with anterior knee pain and patella alta do not respond as well to quadriceps strengthening as patients without patella alta. Nevertheless, surgical distal advancement of the tibial tubercle generally is not recommended because of the difficulty of balancing the patellofemoral articulation and the possibility of increasing patellofemoral contact forces. Nonsurgical stretching of the quadriceps mechanism may be useful.

ANTERIOR CRUCIATE LIGAMENT TEARS

As recently as the 1970s, women who presented with a hemarthrosis, especially after a noncontact injury, were thought to have suffered a patellar dislocation until proven otherwise. Women were "too dainty" to tear their anterior cruciate ligaments (ACLs), and ACL tears were thought to be mostly due to contact injuries, such as those seen in football. As use of the diagnostic arthroscope became more prevalent, it was found that ACL tears could indeed occur from a noncontact mechanism, that they could occur without concomitant medial collateral ligament tears, and they could occur in females. In fact, in recent years, a higher incidence of ACL injuries in females has been noted in team handball,[50] gymnastics,[51] volleyball,[52] alpine skiing,[53] basketball,[54] and soccer.[55] Women have been found to suffer ACL injuries from two to four times as frequently as men engaged in soccer and basketball, respectively.[55] The injury mechanism, however, may be different for men and women. In an NCAA data collection of ACL injuries in soccer, a noncontact mechanism was noted in over half of women's ACL injuries, whereas contact was the primary mechanism of injury in men's ACL injuries. The increased risk of ACL injuries in female athletes is likely multifactorial, and research is ongoing in many different arenas. Some current areas of investigation include an estrogen effect on ligament laxity, deficiencies in training (muscular imbalance, coordination, proprioception),[56] femoral notch width anatomy,[57,58] and shoe-surface interface.

To date, no consistent relationship has been proven between excessive ligamentous laxity and knee injury. Although Nicholas[59] reported that 72% of football players with knee injuries were hypermobile, this has neither been replicated nor substantiated in the female athlete. Furthermore, no conclusive relationship has been found between hypermobility in general, laxity of the knee, and ACL injury.[60]

The size of the femoral intercondylar notch and its role in noncontact ACL tears has been investigated by a number of authors. Souryal and Freeman[57] prospectively studied 902 high school athletes and found that athletes with noncontact ACL injuries had a smaller notch width index (NWI) than athletes whose ACLs tore from a contact mechanism. In addition, they found the mean NWI in females to be smaller than that in males. LaPrade and Burnett,[58] however, studied 213 Division I athletes in several sports and found no significant sex differences in NWI or in the rate of ACL tears. At present, no conclusive evidence exists concerning the roles of notch width, notch width index, and gender in ACL tears. In addition, the relationship of the size of the ACL relative to the size of the intercondylar notch is unknown.

Examination of athletic shoes and shoe-surface interface deserves further research. However, the physician must ponder the increased incidence of ACL injuries in females in two sports with similar mechanics, ie, deceleration, plant, and pivot, but with very different shoe-surface requirements. Soccer is played in a cleated shoe on a field, and basketball is played in an impact-absorbing non-cleated shoe on an indoor court. In a study of team handball in Norway, investigators found that on green turf certain shoes had a higher friction rate, which correlated with a higher incidence of ACL injuries.[61] The role of shoes remains intriguing. After all, male and female anatomy have not changed significantly, whereas there have been marked changes in athletics shoewear.

Skill level and training have been implicated as causative factors in ACL injuries. For example, the recent influx of women into soccer may have decreased the average skill level, strength, and coordination of those playing the sport. Indeed, a survey of Norway Cup soccer tournaments showed a decrease in overall injuries from 32 per week to 17 per week among female players over a 3-year period.[62] Improved skill level was believed to be the likely reason for the decrease. Injury rates for knees in general and ACLs in particular have remained relatively constant over the last 5 years.[55] Further data collection, with a more quantifiable measurement of skill level of the participants, history of sports participation, and matching of skill levels in tournament participants, will help support or dispel the role of skill in ACL injury.

Despite the higher incidence of ACL injuries in female athletes compared with male athletes, an injury to the ACL in the college athlete is still rel-atively infrequent. Extrapolating from the NCAA injury-surveillance data, assuming 15 athletes participate in each basketball practice or game, an ACL injury would occur in one of 952 activity sessions in men, and one of every 247 sessions in women.[63] Because of the numerous benefits sports provide for women as well as men, the increased incidence of ACL injuries in women should not warrant a change in the way women compete or in the sports they choose. Rather, it should stimulate research to examine the multiple variables that may contribute to this difference. Results of such research may contribute to a safer athletic experience for all participants.

History, Physical Examination, and Additional Studies
The findings do not differ from those in the male athlete, nor does the diagnostic testing.

Treatment
There are certain features of the female knee that deserve special consideration when contemplating surgical reconstruction of the ACL. These include the size of the knee, preexisting patellofemoral pain, and ligamentous laxity.

Little is known about the relationship between the size of the ACL, the width of the intercondylar notch, and the width of the distal femur. Souryal and Freeman[57] found that the intercondylar notch in men was wider, not simply because of larger bone structure or larger overall size, but because the notch in men occupied more space in the distal femur than it did in women. Whether this indicated that it also housed a larger ACL was speculated, but was not known. A large graft in a small knee carries with it the potential complication of graft impingement.[64] In addition, if it is harvested from the patella, a large autograft can potentially lead to patellar donor site fracture[64,65] and diminished structural integrity of the remaining patellar tendon.[66]

In addition, there are those who believe that patellar tendon autograft should not be used in women because of the increased chances of postoperative patellofemoral pain.[67] Autogenous patellar bone-tendon-bone is the most commonly used graft source for ACL reconstruction. However, harvesting the patellar tendon disrupts the extensor mechanism, and patellofemoral dysfunction and deficits in quadriceps strength have been reported.[68,69] The morbidity of autogenous patellar tendon harvest is of short duration, however, and the quadriceps weakness is largely reversible when the patient participates in a good rehabilitation program postoperatively.[70,71] Nevertheless, concerns about the extensor mechanism often are cited as reasons for using allograft[72,73] or hamstring autograft,[74,75] especially in patients with preexisting patellofemoral symptoms. In dancers, the surgeon should also use the technique least likely to result in any loss of knee extension because full extension is required aesthetically. With regard to the hypermobile patient, special care should be taken to avoid stretching of the graft after ACL reconstruction in the hyperextended knee.

KNEE PAIN IN THE MASTERS ATHLETE

The masters athlete with knee pain may have osteoarthritis of the patellofemoral joint, a single tibiofemoral compartment, or the entire knee. Degenerative meniscal tears are common. The diagnosis and treatment of these conditions is no different in the female than in the male. However, women who must give up running are more likely than men to find aquarobics or low impact aerobics an acceptable alternative form of aerobic exercise.

THE LEG: EXERTIONAL COMPARTMENT SYNDROME

Exertional compartment syndrome is part of the differential diagnosis of shin splints.[76] Although the clinical picture and diagnosis are no different in the female athlete than in the male athlete, additional etiologic factors in the female athlete may change the treatment options. These etiologic factors are related to the menstrual cycle and to hormonal therapy.

Some female athletes will report that the problem of activity-induced leg pain occurs only during the week preceding their menstrual periods. These are usually ovulatory women who have generalized swelling and fluid retention premenstrually. This baseline fluid retention allows less room for the additional muscle swelling that occurs during exercise, and symptoms of increased compartmental pressure result. Assuming there are no contraindications, women with cyclic symptoms can be treated with oral contraceptives that suppress ovulation and its resultant fluid retention.

Despite a positive response to hormone therapy for the women described above, other women develop exertional compartment syndrome when they use hormonal therapy for contraceptive purposes. These women have no leg symptoms prior to taking oral contraceptives, but the progesterone component of the contraceptive induces fluid retention with resulting activity-related symptoms. These women can be treated either by changing the chemical contraceptive to one containing lower doses of progesterone or by changing to a physical rather than chemical contraceptive method. Because exertional compartment syndrome is potentially treatable in women without resorting to fasciotomy or a change in activity level, it is valuable to ask the female athlete whether she is taking oral contraceptives or whether she has noted any association between her symptoms and the time in her menstrual cycle when they occur.

THE FOOT

MORTON'S NEUROMA

Morton's neuroma is seven to ten times more prevalent in women than in men.[77,78] It is especially problematic in dancers, including aerobic dancers, and in runners. Although originally described in the third web space in the foot, intermetatarsal neuromas can occur in any interspace. They were previously thought more likely to occur in the third interspace because of a junction between the medial and lateral plantar nerves. However, Levitsky and associates[79] found such a junction in only 27% of 71 cadaveric feet and showed that the more common problem was the size of the space between the metatarsal heads. These authors found that the ratio of the digital nerve diameter to the intermetatarsal head distance was significantly smaller in web spaces two and three than in web spaces one and four, accounting for the propensity for neuromata to occur in the second and third web spaces.

The athletes who develop intermetatarsal neuromata spend a disproportionate amount of time bearing weight on their metatarsal heads. Sometimes this is a function of the sport; other times it is related to an anatomic variant, such as a cavus foot or a tight Achilles tendon (often associated with each other).

History and Physical Examination

Patients with intermetatarsal neuromata present with forefoot pain that is made worse when they are doing activities on the balls of their feet or when they are wearing shoes with a narrow forefoot. The pain may radiate into the adjacent toes. Sometimes there is numbness, but this occurs late in the presentation.

On physical examination, there is tenderness to palpation in the involved intermetatarsal space. Exacerbation of pain may be elicited by axial pressure in the involved web space or by squeezing the metatarsal heads laterally. If a click is produced during lateral pressure (Mulder's sign), the neuroma is already fibrotic and is unlikely to respond to nonsurgical care. The physician should test and document sensation in the adjacent toes. He or she should also look for underlying anatomic contributing factors, such as tight Achilles tendons, a cavus foot, or even forefoot varus, which will overload the lateral part of the foot. Many women have a combination of a bunion and a third web space neuroma. In these women, discomfort from the bunion has caused the patient to shift her weight to the lateral side of her foot and produce a neuroma. In this case, treatment of the bunion should also be undertaken to prevent recurrence. The physician should also look for subtle spreading of the toes on either side of the neuroma. This spreading usually implies the presence of either a large neuroma or an associated synovial cyst.[77]

Additional Studies

Plain radiographs may reveal spreading of the metatarsals on either side of the neuroma and can rule out other causes of forefoot pain. Ultrasound and MRI also have been used to diagnose Morton's neuroma with varying degrees of success.[78,80]

Treatment

Initial treatment should include a metatarsal bar or pad proximal to the neuroma. (For athletes who dance barefooted or in soft slippers, the pad can be taped to the foot rather than to the shoe (see "Shoes"). This unweights the area of the neuroma in addition to spreading the metatarsals slightly. The patient should be advised to wear well-padded shoes whenever possible and to make sure that the width of the forepart of the shoe is adequate. Tight Achilles tendons should be stretched. When these treatments fail to produce relief, the neuroma can be injected with a mixture of xylocaine and corticosteroid.[81] Forty-seven percent of patients treated with injection can be expected to obtain relief.[81] To confirm location of the injection, we have the patient wait in the office to see that a digital nerve block has been achieved. Finally, resecting the neuroma from a dorsal approach is successful in relieving symptoms in 90% of patients.[82] Because the proximal cut end of the nerve rounds off into a new neuroma, we make sure that the level of resection is well proximal to the weightbearing region of the metatarsal heads. Postoperatively, to minimize the size of the postoperative neuroma, we also suggest that the patient wear a cushioned shoe, such as a running or aerobic dance shoe, and refrain from activity on the balls of the feet (ie, no dancing or running) for 6 weeks.

FLEXOR HALLUCIS TENDINITIS

Flexor hallucis longus tendinitis is most common in the female ballerina who dances "en pointe" (on the tips of her toes). When the dancer is "en pointe," the flexor hallucis longus acts as an accessory push-off muscle.

History and Physical Examination

The ballerina presents with pain posterior to the medial malleolus, just anterior to the Achilles tendon. The pain is made worse by dancing on the balls of the feet (demi-pointe) or "en pointe." Pain can be elicited by asking the dancer to flex the interphalangeal joint of her great toe against resistance. When a nodule has developed on the tendon, triggering may occur.[83] The distal phalanx is then stuck in flexion until it is passively extended (often with a sudden snap).

Treatment

When trigger toe is not present, the tendinitis is treated with ice massage and nonsteroidal anti-inflammatory drugs (NSAIDs). When nodules are present, the tendon sheath should be opened surgically and the nodules should be removed.

ANKLE IMPINGEMENT

Ankle impingement following an ankle sprain is usually due to impingement on the anterior tibiofibular ligament by an anteriorly subluxating talus,[84] or by a "meniscoid" lesion (scar tissue).[85] However, another type of impingement occurs anteriorly in soccer players and both anteriorly and posteriorly in dancers. Soccer players develop traction osteophytes on the neck of the talus or the tibial plafond or both. These can impinge during ankle dorsiflexion, causing pain and decreased range of motion. In dancers, these osteophytes are more likely to develop in the female ballerina who forces plantarflexion of her foot to dance "en pointe." Other dancers have no osteophytes but suffer from pinching of the synovium of the ankle joint during extremes of dorsiflexion or plantarflexion. When a dancer lands a jump, the ankle must maximally dorsiflex. This dorsiflexion may pinch the anterior synovium and, over time, lead to synovial hypertrophy, which makes further impingement even more likely. Posterior impingement occurs during maximal plantarflexion when the dancer is on the ball of her foot and, especially, on the tips of her toes. A large posterior process of the talus or an os trigonum can add to the impingement posteriorly.[86]

History, Physical Examination, and Additional Studies

The dancer with anterior impingement presents with pain across the anterior aspect of the ankle. Tenderness to ·palpation will be present on the joint line. Swelling may be present and manifest anterolaterally. Pain will be precipitated by forcing dorsiflexion of the ankle, especially while bearing weight. The ˙dancer with posterior impingement presents with pain in the back of the ankle deep to the Achilles tendon. Tenderness to palpation will be present and is easily confused with retrocalcaneal bursitis. Pain will be precipitated by forcing plantarflexion of the ankle.

The physician should obtain radiographs of the ankle. The lateral radiograph should be taken in maximal dorsiflexion to look for anterior impingement and in maximal plantarflexion to look for posterior impingement.

Treatment

When no bony impingement is noted, both anterior and posterior impingement can be treated by using ice and oral NSAIDs. The patient with anterior impingement will benefit from a heel lift in street shoes for about 3 weeks and from avoiding jumps and pliés. Patients with posterior impingement should avoid the plantarflexed position. If no relief is obtained, a single steroid injection into the ankle joint may be helpful. When bony impingement is present, the osteophytes or os trigonum can be removed surgically.[86-88]

POSTERIOR TIBIAL TENDINITIS

The posterior tibial tendon functions to invert the hindfoot and lock the talar joints during heel strike. It also contributes to the maintenance of the longitudinal arch. Stress is put on the posterior tibial tendon during the pronation and the push-off phases of walking and running, especially during sports, such as basketball, soccer, and tennis, that require frequent sudden directional changes. Tendinitis and rupture of the tendon are more prevalent in women, especially in those over the age of 40 years.[89] It is possible to speculate that the higher prevalence of posterior tibial tendon problems in females may be related to the increased prevalence of femoral anteversion, which usually results in compensatory pronation in the foot. The latter is associated with increased hindfoot valgus, which puts the posterior tibial tendon on stretch and may render the retromalleolar part of the tendon relatively avascular.

History and Physical Examination

The patient presents with retromalleolar medial ankle pain that sometimes radiates into the arch. The pain is usually insidious in onset but may have been preceded by minor trauma. Some patients have noted a gradual loss of longitudinal arch. On physical examination, swelling may be noted behind the medial malleolus, and the posterior tibial tendon will be tender on palpation. Asking the patient to plantarflex and invert the foot against resistance may reproduce pain, and stretching the tendon by everting the foot may also produce pain in more inflamed cases. In women with long-standing problems, the physician will see a loss of longitudinal arch, an increase in heel valgus, and abduction of the forefoot. When the patient attempts to stand on her toes, the heel of the affected foot does not invert as it does on the normal side. Total inability to lift the heel off the ground indicates severe dysfunction and probable rupture. Patients with posterior tibial tendon problems should also be examined for tight Achilles tendons, which can cause increased midfoot pronation during push-off.[90]

Additional Studies

Standing anteroposterior (AP) and lateral views of the foot as well as a standing axial view of the calcaneus should be obtained. When the posterior tibial tendon has been deteriorating or torn over time, the radiograph will reveal medial talar displacement on the navicular on the AP view. The lateral view will reveal sagging of the talonavicular and naviculocuneiform joints and loss of the height of the longitudinal arch. The axial view may show increased valgus inclination of the heel. MRI may demonstrate a tear in the posterior tibial tendon or, with the help of "stir" imaging, edema in the tendon sheath.

Treatment

When the posterior tibial tendon is inflamed but seems intact, initial treatment includes rest, ice, NSAIDs, and, most importantly, medial and longitudinal arch support to take the tension off the tendon. Rarely, immobilization will be required to decrease inflammation.

When the swelling and tenderness have decreased, the patient should be taught posterior tibial strengthening exercises using tubing and free weights. If the Achilles tendons are tight, instruction should be given in proper stretching. Often the patient will have been doing Achilles stretching in such a way that a plumb line from the knee falls medial to the ankle (Fig. 28), actually stretching the posterior tibial tendon and not the Achilles. This should be pointed out to the patient and corrected. Patients are more likely to stretch their Achilles correctly if they do so by standing on the edge of a stair and lowering their heels until they feel a stretch. This can also be done on an incline board.

When tendinitis does not respond to nonsurgical treatment, surgical exploration of the tendon between the medial malleolus and the navicular will often reveal synovial proliferation in the tendon sheath. The hypertrophic synovium should be debrided. If a significant degree of degeneration (tendinosis) is noted in the tendon itself, this area should be debrided and the tendon backed up by anastomosing it to the flexor digitorum longus tendon.

In the case of tendon rupture, surgical treatment is generally recommended in the athlete. If foot deformity has not yet occurred, and the site of rupture is retromalleolar, the area of rupture can be repaired primarily and backed up by a

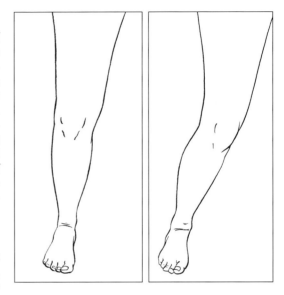

FIGURE 28
Correct (**left**) and incorrect (**right**) methods of stretching the Achilles tendon.

side-to-side anastomosis with the flexor digitorum longus.[91] If the site of the tear is insertional, the tendon is advanced for reinsertion into the navicular bone. When foot deformity has occurred, soft-tissue procedures typically do not suffice. The best treatment in this situation is controversial. Some authors have recommended subtalar arthrodesis, whereas others have recommended calacaneal osteotomy and lateral column lengthening.[92,93] In either case, the foot is immobilized in a nonweightbearing cast for at least 6 weeks, followed by gradually increasing weightbearing with an orthosis.

BUNIONS

Bunions are nine times as common in women as in men, due to a combination of hereditary predisposition, poorly fitting shoewear, ligamentous laxity, and overpronation.[94,95] The last can occur as a result of ligamentous laxity or as a result of compensation for increased femoral anteversion. Overpronation causes increased valgus stress on the great toe during push-off. Bunions also occur in ballet dancers whose first three toes are not of even length, and those whose weight falls medial to the great toe when "en pointe."[96]

History and Physical Examination

Initially the pain from a bunion is limited to the prominent tissue at the medial side of the first metatarsal head. Subsequently, as the great toe drifts into more valgus, and bears less weight, pain can shift to the heads of the second and third metatarsals. Dorsal subluxation of the second toe can cause deformities and corns on the interphalangeal joint as well. In addition to noting the obvious bunion and deviation of the great toe, the physician should also assess the mobility of the first metatarsal and its length relative to the second metatarsal.

Additional Studies

Standing AP and lateral radiographs of both feet should be taken. The physician should note the first and second intermetatarsal angle as well as the relative lengths of these metatarsals. The degree of hallux valgus should be noted. Any metatarsophalangeal arthritis or subluxation of the sesamoids should be recorded.

Treatment

In the athlete, particularly the running athlete, dancer, or gymnast, the treatment of bunions requires attention to certain principles. The goal of treatment is to produce a stable correction while maintaining adequate range of motion of the first metatarsophalangeal joint. Nonsurgical treatment can include padding the forefoot of the athletics shoes. In addition, orthoses, including medial support to decrease the valgus stress and a metatarsal pad to decrease the weight borne on the second and third metatarsal heads, may be helpful. A deep toe box may alleviate symptoms resulting from subluxation of the second toe on top of the first. A shoe with a straighter last will also help to control pronation.

Surgical treatment of bunions should not be performed during the active career of dancers or athletes, such as sprinters or gymnasts, who require extreme dorsiflexion of the first metatarsophalangeal joint. They should be treated symptomatically until their "careers" are over. During surgical treatment, it is particularly important not to interfere with the sesamoids and to avoid dorsal or plantar displacement of the first metatarsal head so that the first metatarsal continues to bear weight appropriately. A chevron osteotomy and bunionectomy have been reported to be successful in elite female runners.[97]

The importance of shoewear fitted to the female athlete cannot be overemphasized. Many women have a wide forefoot and narrow hindfoot and have problems with fit. Women tend to buy shoes to avoid slippage at the heel and may end up with a shoe that is too narrow in the forefoot. Instead, a shoe with a combination last, or a shoe with a variable eyelet pattern that allows adjustable lacing for the forefoot and hindfoot will provide necessary width in the forefoot and a snug fit in the hindfoot (see "Shoes").

REFERENCES

1. Fulkerson JP: Patellofemoral pain disorders: Evaluation and management. *J Am Acad Orthop Surg* 1994;2:124-132.

2. DeHaven KE, Lintner DM: Athletic injuries: Comparison by age, sport, and gender. *Am J Sports Med* 1986;14:218-224.

3. Muneta T, Yamamoto H, Ishibashi T, et al: Computerized tomographic analysis of tibial tubercle position in the painful female patellofemoral joint. *Am J Sports Med* 1994; 22:67-71.

4. Ogden JA: The uniqueness of growing bones, in Rockwood CA Jr, Wilkins KE, King RE (eds): *Fractures in Children.* Philadelphia, PA, JB Lippincott, 1984, vol 3, pp 1-86.

5. Tanner JM (ed): *Growth at Adolescence, With a General Consideration of the Effects of Hereditary and Environmental Factors Upon Growth and Maturation From Birth to Maturity,* ed 2. Oxford, England, Blackwell Scientific, 1962.

6. Atwater AE: Biomechanics and the female athlete, in Puhl JL, Brown CH, Voy RO (eds): *Sports Science Perspectives for Women.* Champaign, IL, Human Kinetics Books, 1988, pp 1-12.

7. Staheli LT: Rotational problems of the lower extremities. *Orthop Clin North Am* 1987; 18:503-512.

8. Staheli LT: Rotational problems in children. *J Bone Joint Surg* 1993;75A:939-949.

9. Hvid I, Andersen LI: The quadriceps angle and its relation to femoral torsion. *Acta Orthop Scand* 1982;53:577-579.

10. Nagamine R, Otani T, White SE, et al: Patellar tracking measurement in the normal knee. *J Orthop Res* 1995;13:115-122.

11. Huberti HH, Hayes WC: Patellofemoral contact pressures: The influence of q-angle and tendo-femoral contact. *J Bone Joint Surg* 1984; 66A:715-724

12. van Kampen A, Huiskes R: The three-dimensional tracking pattern of the human patella. *J Orthop Res* 1990;8:372-382.

13. James SL: Chondromalacia of the patella in the adolescent, in Kennedy JC, Fowler PT (eds): *The Injured Adolescent Knee.* Baltimore, MD, Williams & Wilkins, 1979, pp 205-251.

14. Laurin CA, Levesque HP, Dussault R, et al: The abnormal lateral patellofemoral angle: A diagnostic roentgenographic sign of recurrent patellar subluxation. *J Bone Joint Surg* 1978; 60A:55-60.

15. Fulkerson JP, Hungerford DS (eds): Patellar tilt/compression and the excessive lateral pressure syndrome (ELPS), in *Disorders of the Patellofemoral Joint,* ed 2. Baltimore, MD, Williams & Wilkins, 1990, pp 102-123.

16. Sage FP: Cerebral palsy, in Crenshaw AH (ed): *Campbell's Operative Orthopaedics.* St Louis, MO, CV Mosby, 1987, p 2876.

17. Ober FR: The role of the iliotibial band and fascia lata as a factor in the causation of low back disabilities and sciatica. *J Bone Joint Surg* 1936; 18A:105-110.

18. Inoue M, Shino K, Hirose H, et al: Subluxation of the patella: Computed tomography analysis of patellofemoral congruence. *J Bone Joint Surg* 1988;70A:1331-1337.

19. Kujala UM, Osterman K, Kormano M, et al: Patello femoral relationships in recurrent patellar dislocation. *Radiology* 1990;175:886-887.

20. Beighton P, Grahame R, Bird H: Clinical features of hypermobility (locomotor system and extra-articular), in *Hypermobility of Joints.* Berlin, Germany, Springer-Verlag, 1983, pp 45-60.

21. Merchant AC, Mercer RL, Jacobsen RH, et al: Roentgenographic analysis of patellofemoral congruence. *J Bone Joint Surg* 1974; 56A:1391-1396.

22. Schutzer SF, Ramsby GR, Fulkerson JP: Computed tomographic classification of patellofemoral pain patients. *Orthop Clin North Am* 1986;17:235-248.

23. Koskinen SK, Taimela S, Nelimarkka O, et al: Magnetic resonance imaging of patellofemoral relationships. *Skeletal Radiol* 1993;22:403-410.

24. Shellock FG, Mink JH, Deutsch AL, et al: Patellar tracking abnormalities: Clinical experience with kinematic MR imaging in 130 patients. *Radiology* 1989;172:799-804.

25. Doucette SA, Goble EM: The effect of exercise on patellar tracking in lateral patellar compression syndrome. *Am J Sports Med* 1992;20: 434-440.

26. O'Neill DB, Micheli LJ, Warner JP: Patellofemoral stress: A prospective analysis of exercise treatment in adolescents and adults. *Am J Sports Med* 1992;20:151-156.

27. Shea KP, Fulkerson JP: Patellofemoral joint injuries, in Griffin LY (ed): *Rehabilitation of the Injured Knee,* ed 2. St. Louis, MO, Mosby Year Book, 1995, pp 121-133.

28. Molnar TJ: Patellofemoral rehabilitaton, in Fox JM, Del Pizzo W (eds): *The Patellofemoral Joint.* New York, NY, McGraw-Hill, 1993, pp 291-304.

29. Stokes M, Young A: Investigations of quadriceps inhibition: Implications for clinical practice. *Physiotherapy* 1984;70:425-428.

30. Olerud C, Berg P: The variation of the Q angle with different positions of the foot. *Clin Orthop* 1984;191:162-165.

31. Steinkamp LA, Dillingham MF, Markel MD, et al: Biomechanical considerations in patellofemoral joint rehabilitation. *Am J Sports Med* 1993;21: 438-444.

32. Werner S, Arvidsson H, Arvidsson I, et al: Electrical stimulation of vastus medialis and stretching of lateral thigh muscles in patients with patello-femoral symptoms. *Knee Surg Sports Traumatol Arthrosc* 1993;1:85-92.

33. McConnell J: The management of chondromalacia patellae: A long term solution. *Austral J Physiother* 1986;32:215-223.

34. Podesta L, Sherman MF: Knee bracing. *Orthop Clin North Am* 1988;19:737-745.

35. Souza DR, Gross MT: Comparison of vastus medialis obliquus:vastus lateralis muscle integrated electromyographic ratios between healthy subjects and patients with patellofemoral pain. *Phys Ther* 1991;71:319-320.

36. Bennett JG, Stauber WT: Evaluation and treatment of anterior knee pain using eccentric exercise. *Med Sci Sport Exerc* 1986;18:526-530.

37. Fulkerson JP, Cautilli RA: Chronic patellar instability: Subluxation and dislocation, in Fox JM, Del Pizzo W (eds): *The Patellofemoral Joint.* New York, NY, McGraw-Hill, 1993, pp 135-147.

38. Takai S, Sakakida K, Yamashita F, et al: Rotational alignment of the lower limb in osteoarthritis of the knee. *Int Orthop* 1985;9: 209-215.

39. Vizsolyi P, Taunton J, Robertson G, et al: Breaststroker's knee: An analysis of epidemiological and biomechanical factors. *Am J Sports Med* 1987;15:63-71.

40. Teitz CC: Dance, in Griffin LY (ed): *Rehabilitation of the Injured Knee,* ed 2. St. Louis, MO, CV Mosby, pp 274-282.

41. Larsen E, Lauridsen F: Conservative treatment of patellar dislocations: Influence of evident factors on the tendency to redislocation and the therapeutic result. *Clin Orthop* 1982;171:131-136.

42. Halbrecht JL, Jackson DW: Malalignment: Acute dislocation of the patella, in Fox JM, Del Pizzo W (eds): *The Patellofemoral Joint.* New York, NY, McGraw-Hill, 1993, pp 123-134.

43. Harilainen A, Myllynen P: Operative treatment in acute patella dislocation: Radiologic predisposing factors, diagnosis and results. *Am J Knee Surg* 1988;1:178.

44. Gilbert TJ, Johnson E, Detlie T, et al: Radiologic case study: Patellar dislocation. Medial retinacular tears, avulsion fractures, and osteochondral fragments. *Orthopedics* 1993;16:732-736.

45. Virolainen H, Visuri T, Kuusela T: Acute dislocation of the patella: MR findings. *Radiology* 1993;189:243-246.

46. Kirsch MD, Fitzgerald SW, Friedman H, et al: Transient lateral patellar dislocation: Diagnosis with MR imaging. *Am J Roentgenol* 1993;161: 109-113.

47. Cash JD, Hughston JC: Treatment of acute patellar dislocation. *Am J Sports Med* 1988;16:244-249.

48. Madigan R, Wissinger HA, Donaldson WF: Preliminary experience with a method of quadricepsplasty in recurrent subluxation of the patella. *J Bone Joint Surg* 1975;57A:600-607.

49. Cox JS: Evaluation of the Roux-Elmslie-Trillat procedure for knee extensor realignment. *Am J Sports Med* 1982;10:303-310.

50. Strand T, Tvedte R, Engebretsen L, et al: Anterior cruciate ligament injuries in handball playing: Mechanisms and incidence of injuries. *Tidsskr Nor Laegeforen* 1990;110:2222-2225.

51. *NCAA injury surveillance system 1992-1993.* Overland Park, KS, National Collegiate Athletic Association.

52. Ferretti A, Papandrea P, Conteduca F, et al: Knee ligament injuries in volleyball players. *Am J Sports Med* 1992;20:203-207.

53. Barber FA: Snow skiing combined anterior cruciate ligament/medial collateral ligament disruptions. *Arthroscopy* 1994;10:85-89.

54. Ireland ML, Wall C: Epidemiology and comparison of knee injuries in elite male and female United States basketball athletes. *Med Sci Sports* 1990;22:592.

55. Arendt E, Dick R: Knee injury patterns among men and women in collegiate basketball and soccer: NCAA data and review of literature. *Am J Sports Med* 1995;23:694-701.

56. Huston LJ, Wojtys EM: Neuromuscular performance characteristics in elite female athletes. *Am J Sports Med* 1996;24:427-436.

57. Souryal TO, Freeman TR: Intercondylar notch size and anterior cruciate ligament injuries in athletes: A prospective study. *Am J Sports Med* 1993;21:535-539.

58. LaPrade RF, Burnett QM II: Femoral intercondylar notch stenosis and correlation to anterior cruciate ligament injuries: A prospective study. *Am J Sports Med* 1994;22:198-203.

59. Nicholas JA: Injuries to knee ligaments: Relationship to looseness and tightness in football players. *JAMA* 1970;212:2236-2239.

60. Harner CD, Paulos LE, Greenwald AE, et al: Detailed analysis of patients with bilateral anterior cruciate ligament injuries. *Am J Sports Med* 1994;22:37-43.

61. Myklebust G, Engebretsen L, Strand T, et al: Abstract: Registration of ACL-injuries in the 3 upper divisions in Norwegian team handball: A prospective study. *Med Sci Sports Exerc* 1993;25:S50.

62. Engebretsen L: Soccer injuries in Norway. *Tidsskr Nor Laegeforen* 1985;105:1766-1769.

63. *NCAA participation study 1989-1990, 1992-1993.* Overland Park, KS, National Collegiate Athletic Association.

64. Cooper DE, Deng XH, Burstein AL, et al: The strength of the central third patellar tendon graft: A biomechanical study. *Am J Sports Med* 1993;21:818-824.

65. McCarroll JR: Fracture of the patella during a golf swing following reconstruction of the anterior cruciate ligament: A case report. *Am J Sports Med* 1983;11:26-27.

66. Burks RT, Haut RC, Lancaster RL: Biomechanical and histological observations of the dog patellar tendon after removal of its central one-third. *Am J Sports Med* 1990;18:146-153.

67. Sachs RA, Daniel DM, Stone ML, et al: Patellofemoral problems after anterior cruciate ligament reconstruction. *Am J Sports Med* 1989;17:760-765.

68. Shelbourne KD, Rubinstein RA Jr, VanMeter CD, et al: Correlation of remaining patellar tendon width with quadriceps strength after autogenous bone-patellar tendon-bone anterior cruciate ligament reconstruction. *Am J Sports Med* 1994;22:774-778.

69. Hughston JC: Complications of anterior cruciate ligament surgery. *Orthop Clin North Am* 1985;16:237-240.

70. Lephart SM, Kocher MS, Harner CD, et al: Quadriceps strength and functional capacity after anterior cruciate ligament reconstruction: Patellar tendon autograft versus allograft. *Am J Sports Med* 1993;21:738-743.

71. Rubinstein RA Jr, Shelbourne KD, VanMeter CD, et al: Isolated autogenous bone-patellar-tendon-bone graft site morbidity. *Am J Sports Med* 1994;22:324-327.

72. Meyers JF: Allograft reconstruction of the anterior cruciate ligament. *Clin Sports Med* 1991;10:487-498.

73. Shino K, Inoue M, Horibe S, et al: Reconstruction of the anterior cruciate ligament using allogeneic tendon: Long-term followup. *Am J Sports Med* 1990;18:457-465.

74. Pagnani MJ, Warner JJ, O'Brien SJ, et al: Anatomic considerations in harvesting the semitendinosus and gracilis tendons and a technique of harvest. *Am J Sports Med* 1993;21:565-571.

75. Sgaglione NA, Warren RF, Wickiewicz TL, et al: Primary repair with semitendinosus tendon augmentation of acute anterior cruciate ligament injuries. *Am J Sports Med* 1990;18:64-73.

76. Hutchinson MR, Ireland M: Common compartment syndromes in athletes: Treatment and rehabilitation. *Sports Med* 1994;17:200-208.

77. Mann RA, Reynolds JC: Interdigital neuroma: A critical clinical analysis. *Foot Ankle* 1983;3:238-243.

78. Shapiro PP, Shapiro SL: Sonographic evaluation of interdigital neuromas. *Foot Ankle Int* 1995;16:604-606.

79. Levitsky KA, Alman BA, Jevsevar DS, et al: Digital nerves of the foot: Anatomic variations and implications regarding the pathogenesis of interdigital neuroma. *Foot Ankle* 1993;14:208-214.

80. Resch S, Stenström A, Jonsson A, et al: The diagnostic efficacy of magnetic resonance imaging and ultrasonograpohy in Morton's neuroma: A radiological-surgical correlation. *Foot Ankle Int* 1994;15:88-92.

81. Bennett GL, Graham CR, Mauldin DM: Morton's interdigital neuroma: A comprehensive treatment protocol. *Foot Ankle Int* 1995;16:760-763.

82. Keh RA, Ballew KK, Higgins KR, et al: Long-term follow-up of Morton's neuroma. *J Foot Surg* 1992;31:93-95.

83. Hamilton WG: Stenosing tenosynovitis of the flexor hallucios longus tendon and posterior impingement upon the os trigonum in ballet dancers. *Foot Ankle* 1982;3:74-80.

84. Bassett FH III, Gates HS III, Billys JB, et al: Talar impingement by the anterior tibiofibular ligament: A cause of chronic pain in the ankle after inversion sprain. *J Bone Joint Surg* 1990;72A:55-59.

85. Ferkel RD, Karzel RP, Del Pizzo W, et al: Arthroscopic treatment of anterolateral impingement of the ankle. *Am J Sports Med* 1991; 19:440-446.

86. Marotta JJ, Micheli LJ: Os trigonum impingement in dancers. *Am J Sports Med* 1992;20:533-536.

87. Kleiger B: Anterior tibiotalar impingement syndrome in dancers. *Foot Ankle* 1982;3:69-73.

88. Jaivin JS, Ferkel RD: Arthroscopy of the foot and ankle. *Clin Sports Med* 1994;3:761-781.

89. Frey CC, Shereff MJ: Tendon injuries about the ankle in athletes. *Clin Sports Med* 1988; 7:103-118.

90. Warren BL: Anatomical factors associated with predicting plantar fasciitis in long distance runners. *Med Sci Sports Exerc* 1984;16:60-63.

91. Mann RA, Thompson FM: Rupture of the posterior tibial tendon causing flatfoot: Surgical treatment. *J Bone Joint Surg* 1985;67A:556-561.

92. Frankel JP, Turf RM, Kuzmicki LM: Double calcaneal osteotomy in the treatment of posterior tibial tendon dysfunction,. *J Foot Ankle Surg* 1995;34:254-261.

93. Resnick RB, Jahss MH, Choueka J, et al: Deltoid ligament forces after tibialis posterior tendon rupture: Effects of triple arthrodesis and calcaneal displacement osteotomies. *Foot Ankle Int* 1995;16:14-20.

94. Hunter-Griffin LY (ed): Female athletes, in *Athletic Training and Sports Medicine,* ed 2. Park Ridge, IL, American Academy of Orthopaedic Surgeons, 1991, pp 921-932.

95. Frey C, Thompson F, Smith J, et al: American Orthopaedic Foot and Ankle Society women's shoe survey. *Foot Ankle* 1993;14:78-81.

96. Teitz CC, Harrington RM, Wiley H: Pressures on the foot in pointe shoes. *Foot Ankle* 1985;5:216-221.

97. Lillich JS, Baxter DE: Bunionectomies and related surgery in the elite female middle-distance and marathon runner. *Amer J Sports Med* 1986;14:491-493.

SHOES

CAROL FREY, MD

Because shoes are a key piece of equipment for many sports, they play a critical role in performance and in injury prevention. If the shoe does not fit and is not properly designed for the sport, not only will the athlete suffer foot injuries, but she will not be able to perform at her best.

It has only been since 1970 that a large number of sport shoes specifically designed for women have been manufactured. Before 1970, golf shoes were one of the few specialty sport shoes made specifically for women. It was recently reported that in 1994, women aged 12 years and older purchased $5.4 billion in athletic footwear, compared with $5.3 billion in footwear purchased by men.[1] Some predict that the women's athletics shoe market will become a battleground for the industry's top competitors. However, even though athletics shoe manufacturers have relied on scientific research, prior experience, and the desire of all those involved in sports to improve performance in the development of their products, little attention has been paid to the specific needs of the female athlete.

FEMALE ANATOMY

In addition to the male and female lower extremity anatomic variations noted in the previous chapter, the female foot generally has a smaller Achilles tendon, has a narrower heel in relationship to the forefoot, and is narrower overall relative to length than a man's foot. Women complete the heel-to-toe gait in a shorter amount of time than men because women's feet are shorter. Furthermore, because leg length in women is 51.2% of total body height compared with 56% in men,[2] women must strike the ground more often to cover the same distance.

Therefore, the cumulative ground reaction forces may be greater in the female runner.

In some studies, elite women runners have been shown to be predominantly midfoot strikers.[3] Only minor differences were found, however, between ground reaction forces in their racing and training shoes. In addition, more abduction during foot placement and greater rear foot motion have also been noted in women runners.[3]

SHOE ANATOMY

THE LAST

The last is considered by many to be the foundation of shoe production and development (Fig. 29). It is a three-dimensional form on which the shoe is made. The last determines the shape and fit of a shoe, including the shape of the toe box, instep, girth, and foot curvature. The largest last variations occur in the girth (or widest part of the forefoot) and in the heel width. When female athletes complain about the difficulty of finding a comfortable athletics shoe, it is usually the last that is to blame. Many women's athletics shoes are simply smaller versions of men's shoes. In these cases, the women's athletics shoe is built on a scaled-down version of a male last rather than on a last based on the anatomy of the female foot. Typically, manufacturers scale down in fixed proportions all key internal dimensions of the men's athletics shoe when making a women's athletics shoe. This process is called scaling or grading. It still is practiced today in the manufacture of many women's athletics shoes, although most major athletics shoe companies now have women's divisions, and many have recently developed anatomic female lasts.

This chapter has been adapted in part from Lutter LD, Mizel MS, Pfeffer GB (eds): *Orthopaedic Knowledge Update: Foot and Ankle*. Rosemont, IL, American Academy of Orthopaedic Surgeons, 1994.

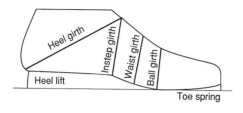

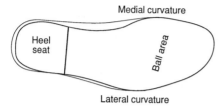

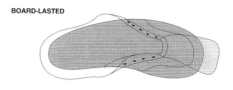

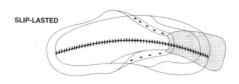

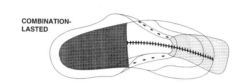

FIGURE 29

The last is a form on which the shoe is made and is thought by many to be the foundation for shoe production, development, and fit. (Reproduced with permission from Lutter LD, Mizel MS, Pfeffer GB (eds): *Orthopaedic Knowledge Update: Foot and Ankle.* Rosemont, IL, American Academy of Orthopaedic Surgeons, 1994, pp 73-88.)

Because most feet have a slight inward curve, most sport-shoe companies use a last that is curved inward approximately 7°. The greater the curve of the last, the greater the foot motion that is allowed. Curved lasts are better suited for female athletes with high arches who do not overpronate. These shoes offer less medial support but more foot mobility. Furthermore, curved lasts are desirable for a faster runner who wants a more responsive shoe. Straight lasts provide more support to the medial side of the foot and are better suited for female athletes with low arches or those who overpronate. Because women tend to pronate somewhat more than men, they may require a straighter last. A combination last is any last that varies from a standard proportional last to accommodate a combination of movement and fit requirements.

LASTING TECHNIQUES

The most common lasting techniques are slip lasting, board (flat) lasting, and combination lasting (Fig. 30). A slip-lasted shoe is constructed by sewing the upper like a moccasin and then gluing it to the sole. The last is usually forced into the upper, which then takes on the shape of the last. A sock liner usually replaces the insole. This lasting method creates a flexible, lightweight shoe with little torsional rigidity.

FIGURE 30

Top, Board last. **Center,** Slip last. **Bottom,** Combination last. (Reproduced with permission from Lutter LD, Mizel MS, Pfeffer GB (eds): *Orthopaedic Knowledge Update: Foot and Ankle.* Rosemont, IL, American Academy of Orthopaedic Surgeons, 1994, pp 73-88.)

When the flat, or board lasting method is used, the upper is placed over the last and attached to the insole with cement, staples, or tacks. This construction provides stability and torsional rigidity, but less flexibility, and provides more pronation control for the heavier or pregnant athlete. Combination lasting is the method used when more than one lasting technique is needed on the same shoe. The usual combination is a shoe that is board-lasted in the heel for stability, but slip-lasted in the forefoot for flexibility.

THE OUTER SOLE

The outer sole, or outsole, is the part of the shoe that makes contact with the ground. It usually is attached to a midsole to form a complete sole. Most outer soles are made of hard carbon rubber or blown rubber compounds. Blown rubber is the lightest outsole material, but carbon rubber is more durable. Many outsoles are composed of both blown and carbon rubber. Blown rubber is used in the forefoot and midfoot and carbon rubber is used in the high impact area of the heel.

TABLE 7

OUTSOLE DESIGN OPTIONS

Design	Type of Shoe
Suction cup	Court
Herringbone	Court
Pivot point	Court
Radial edge	Court
Multiclaw (stud)	Field
Asymmetric stud	Field
Traction and wear lug	Hiking and climbing (boots)
Cantilevered (for shock absorption)	Running
Wear area reinforcement	Running

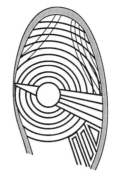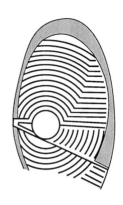

FIGURE 31

Outsole patterns with a concentric circle pattern and radiating lines for the purpose of forefoot flexion. These outsole patterns typically are seen in basketball shoes. (Reproduced with permission from Lutter LD, Mizel MS, Pfeffer GB (eds): *Orthopaedic Knowledge Update: Foot and Ankle.* Rosemont, IL, American Academy of Orthopaedic Surgeons, 1994, pp 73-88.)

Other materials used in the outer sole include gum rubbers, which are hard-wearing and grip well on most surfaces, and polyurethane (PU), which is durable but less versatile as an outsole material. Nylon, leather, and polyvinyl chloride have outsole applications for specific sports.

Patterns in the outer sole can enhance stability and traction.[4] Cutouts and patterns can also eliminate weight in the shoe by exposing the middle part of the midsole. The design of the outsole can provide traction, cushioning, pivot points, flexpaths, and wear plugs. Outsoles are designed for specific sports, weather conditions, and surfaces (Table 7) (Fig. 31).

The traction provided by the outsole is an important aspect in the design of a sport shoe and is directly related to the ability of the shoe to develop frictional forces with the playing surface. The traction needs depend on the specific sport. A balance must be reached between too little traction, which may have a negative effect on athletic performance, and too much traction, which may put the athlete at risk for injury. The traction needs of the female athlete do not differ significantly from the needs of the male athlete.

THE MIDSOLE AND HEEL WEDGE

Many of the recent advances in the athletics shoe industry have been made in midsole materials and design. The midsole and heel wedge are located between the shoe's upper and the outsole, attaching to both. These components provide shock absorption, lift, cushioning, and control. The female athlete completes the heel-to-toe gait faster than the male, and because she has a shorter leg length and her feet must strike the ground more often to cover the same distance, her cushioning needs may actually be greater than the male athlete's. In addition, the midsole must have the ability to control pronation. This control is an important feature of any women's athletics shoe.

The midsole is manufactured from a combination of two basic materials: ethyl vinyl acetate (EVA) and PU. EVA is lightweight, has excellent cushioning properties, and is available in various densities. PU is a heavier, denser, and more durable material than EVA; however, new forms of lighter PU are being developed. The firmest densities in a multidensity midsole are usually represented by a darker color. These can be placed at specific points in the midsole to aid in motion control. Both EVA and PU are used to encapsulate other cushioning materials such as gel, air bags, silicone, and honeycomb pads.

OTHER SHOE COMPONENTS

The Tongue

The tongue is designed primarily to protect the dorsum of the foot from moisture, dirt, and lace pressure. Lacing loops or tongue slits help prevent the tongue from slipping.

The Toe Box

The toe box is made up of a stiff material that is inserted between the lining and the upper in the toe area to protect the toes. There should be ample room in the toe box to prevent development of, or symptoms from, bunions, hammertoes, corns, calluses, and neuromas.

Sock Linings, Arch Supports, and Inserts

The sock lining covers the insole and improves comfort and appearance. A prime function of the sock lining is to serve as an interface between the shoe and the foot. Sock linings are molded, soft support systems that function in moisture absorption, aeration, hygiene, shock absorption, and motion control.

Custom molded "foothotics" have been made popular by the ski industry. These semirigid insole devices are custom molded to the foot and may help increase comfort, shock absorption, and performance. Custom insoles can be used in any sport shoe provided there is enough room to accommodate the insert. They are most commonly used in shoes for the female athlete to prevent hyperpronation.

Heel Counters

The heel counter is a firm cup, built into the rear of the shoe, that holds the heel in position and helps control excessive hindfoot motion. Most heel counters today are made of a durable plastic such as stytherm, thermoplastic, or polyvinyl. The medial side of the heel counter may be extended or reinforced for additional pronation control in the female athlete. Contoured or notched counters also reduce irritation of the Achilles tendon that can occur in plantarflexion. They may be slightly smaller in women's athletics shoes to accommodate the smaller Achilles tendon.

Foxing

Foxing is a stripping material, usually made of suede or rubber, that provides medial and lateral support to the outside of the shoe. In running shoes, the most important foxing is at the toe and is called the toe cap. In court shoes, the foxing runs completely around the sole for lateral support.

NEW COMPONENTS AND DESIGNS

Air Systems

Air systems, which were first introduced in 1979, use encapsulated air units in the midsole to enhance cushioning. Ambient air or freon also can be used. Depending on the model, the air units may be in the heel, forefoot, or both. Initial reports noted that although air systems had superior shock absorption, their stability was poor.[5] Stability in the context of sports refers to the ability of the shoe to resist excessive or unwanted motion of the foot and ankle. Shoes with very soft, well-cushioned midsoles allow significantly more motion than firmer shoes, and a poor design can be unstable. Air systems are not as susceptible to compaction as EVA, PU, and other midsole materials; therefore, they are thought to be more durable.

Pronation-Control Devices

Controlling overpronation in runners and other female athletes is a major concern of the athletics shoe industry. Most of the motion-control features that limit or control pronation fall into one of two categories: a harder density material that is built into the medial aspect of the midsole and/or heel, or a medial component that is to the inside or outside of the shoe. In the past, most of the pronation-control devices have focused on controlling the rear foot. More attention is now being placed on controlling the entire foot.

SHOE FIT

Many women complain about the difficulty of finding a comfortable athletics shoe.[6] As mentioned above, a shoe's fit depends largely on the shape of the three-dimensional last used to form it, and many women's athletics shoes are simply scaled down versions of the men's athletics shoes. However, the female foot has a different shape from the male foot. In general, it is narrower relative to length, with a narrower heel compared to the forefoot. As the foot length increases, forefoot width increases somewhat, but heel width does not increase significantly, especially in feet larger than size seven. Yet, as shoe length increases, manufacturers typically scale the shoes by enlarging all the key internal dimensions in fixed proportions. The result is often shoes that are too loose in the hindfoot.

Because the shape of the shoe should match the shape of the athlete's foot, female athletes often have difficulty obtaining a proper shoe fit. One recent study indicated that 88% of women were wearing shoes that were smaller in width than their feet, and, as a result, they were suffering from painful foot deformities.[7] Women with bigger feet (size eight and larger) had more pain and deformity than women with smaller feet. This group of women may have had a more difficult time with shoe fit than the women with smaller feet. In their cases, the heel counters of the larger shoes may not have gripped the heel, and a smaller shoe size was selected. Although the smaller shoe would have provided the proper heel fit, it may have been too snug for the forefoot, which could have resulted in deformity and pain. These women would require a combination last for proper shoe fit.

Shoes should feel comfortable and fit well the first time they are put on. Runners and other athletes should shop for shoes after a run or training session, when their feet are at their largest. The shoe should be fit to the largest foot. A recent study of 356 women indicated that 66% of them had one foot that was larger than the other.[7] When the shoe is being fit, there should be a finger's breadth from the end of the toe box to the end of the longest toe, and the athlete should be able to fully extend all toes.

Although the most common regular shoe width is C for men and B for women, the average athletics shoe width is D for men and C for women. This reflects additional allowances for foot expansion and movement during sport. Width fittings are not commonly available in athletics footwear. Athletics shoes are generally built on "universal" or male lasts, and width adjustments are incorporated into lacing patterns.

When fitting new shoes, the athlete should wear the socks normally used while training. If the athlete normally wears orthoses, these should replace the sock liner of the shoe during fitting. Using different lacing patterns can help the female athlete fine tune the fit of her shoe.

LACES

To provide a more comfortable shoe fit and distribute stress evenly across the dorsum of the foot, laces should be pulled and tightened one set of eyelets at a time. Lacing should begin at the bottom of the shoe. The majority of athletes can use the conventional criss-cross pattern of lacing to achieve a snug but comfortable fit. However, there are many lacing patterns (Fig. 32) and shoe manufacturers have added extra eyelets so athletes can lace their shoes for a custom fit.

Many sport shoes incorporate variable-width or dual lacing systems. These provide a variable eyelet pattern that allows conventional lacing to be adjusted for variation in foot size. Female athletes who are having a difficult time with shoe fit should look for shoes designed with these features. The wider placed eyelets allow the lacing

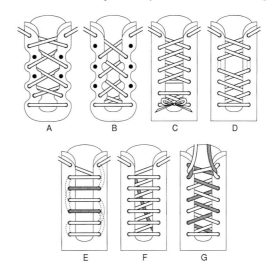

FIGURE 32

Lacing patterns. (**A**) Variable width lacing for narrow fitting. (**B**) Variable width lacing for wide fitting. (**C**) Independent lacing system using two laces. (**D**) Criss-cross alternative pattern to avoid a dorsal prominence or painful area. (**E**) Lacing pattern recommended for high arches. Note that the laces never cross over the top of the foot. (**F**) Lacing pattern that pulls the toe box of the shoe up, relieving pressure on the toes. Weave the lace from the inside front eyelet to the opposite last eyelet. (**G**) Criss-cross and loop lacing system holds the foot snugly in the shoe. This pattern is recommended for all athletes with heel blisters or the female athlete with heel slippage. (Reproduced with permission from Lutter LD, Mizel MS, Pfeffer GB (eds): *Orthopaedic Knowledge Update: Foot and Ankle.* Rosemont, IL, American Academy of Orthopaedic Surgeons, 1994, pp 73-88.)

to pull the quarters in more tightly for narrow feet. The narrower placed eyelets allow for more width and are thus more suitable for a wider foot.

LACING TECHNIQUES

In an independent lacing system, one lace is provided for the proximal eyelets and a second one is provided for the distal eyelets, which can be tied at different tensions for a custom fit. Many females with a relatively wide forefoot compared to their hindfoot find this pattern useful.

Another lacing pattern can relieve pressure over a dorsal prominence and painful areas of the foot. If the athlete experiences dorsal pain or nerve entrapment, she starts with a conventional lacing system until just distal to the problem area. The lace is then moved vertically to the next eyelet so it does not cross over the dorsum of the foot. A conventional lacing pattern is used to complete the closure.

The square box lacing technique distributes lace pressure more evenly over the dorsum of the foot than does the criss-cross lacing system. In this method, the laces never cross over the dorsum of the foot but rather pass under the eyelet. This is useful for a female athlete with a high arch, rigid feet, or a dorsal prominence.

The single lace cross technique may help the athlete who is having problems with black or sore toenails. One lace runs from the inside most proximal eyelet to the opposite most distal eyelet. The other end of the lace goes side to side through the remaining eyelets. This pattern pulls the toe box off the toes to relieve pressure. Female tennis players and athletes with bunions, hammertoes, or corns find this pattern useful.

A technique to help prevent heel slippage, a common problem in the female athlete, consists of a conventional lacing pattern until the last eyelet is reached. By looping the end of each lace and using the loop as an eyelet, a more secure pull on the laces is achieved.

ELASTIC LACES

Elastic laces can be beneficial to the female athlete with wide or expanding feet; however, shoes will lose some stability because as the foot rolls in, the laces will give. The elastic lace eliminates the need for lacelocks used by many triathletes because the extra stretch allows shoes to be pulled on easily. These laces sometimes are useful for the pregnant athlete.

SPORT SPECIFIC SHOES

Athletics shoes are grouped by the manufacturers into seven sales categories (Table 8).

TABLE 8

SALES CATEGORIES OF ATHLETICS SHOES AS GROUPED BY MANUFACTURERS

Category	Type of Sport
Running, training, and walking shoes	Walking and running
Court sport shoes	Court
Field sport shoes	Field
Winter sport shoes	Skiing, skating, all other winter sports
Outdoor sport shoes	Hunting, fishing, boating, other similar recreational sports
Track and field shoes	Track and field
Specialty sport shoes	Golf, aerobic exercise, other specialized sports

RUNNING, TRAINING, AND WALKING SHOES

Running, training, and walking shoes are used for hiking, race walking, and exercise walking.

Running Spikes

Little body weight is placed on the heel in sprinting. For most track runners, even those who run the longer distances, landing and propulsion are carried out on the fore and middle part of the foot. For this reason, track shoes used in the faster and shorter races have just enough padding at the heel to prevent a contusion (Fig. 33).

A slight wedge in the shoes for longer races gives more torsional rigidity and support. Torsional rigidity is often omitted in track shoes for lightness. Track shoe lasts are designed to hug the foot at the heel, waist, and ball of the shoe. The toe box is semipointed to prevent the toes from splaying during landing and takeoff.

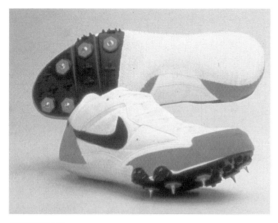

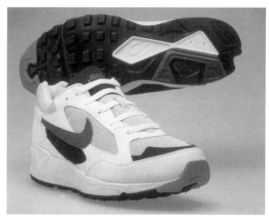

FIGURE 33

Spikes have just enough padding in the heel to prevent a contusion. The toe box is semipointed and the shoe contains a maximum of six sole and two heel spikes. (Reproduced with permission from NIKE. Any illustrations of or statements about commercial products are solely the opinion(s) of the author(s) and do not represent an Academy endorsement or evaluation of these products.)

FIGURE 34

The features of a good running shoe include cushioning, flexibility, control, and stability in the heel counter area, torsional rigidity in the waist or shank, lightness, comfort, traction, motion control, and good fit. (Reproduced with permission from NIKE. Any illustrations of or statements about commercial products are solely the opinion(s) of the author(s) and do not represent an Academy endorsement or evaluation of these products.)

There are certain specifications for track spikes, with some variability for different events. A maximum of six sole and two heel spikes is permitted. Spikes must not project more than 25 mm or exceed 4 mm in diameter. Added spike receptacles may be present for adjustment and may be filled with flat screws when not in use. Grooves, ridges, and appendages are permitted on the sole and heel. For use on synthetic and rubber tracks, track spikes have been shortened to project approximately 9 mm. A total of six spikes allows better traction. With the shorter spikes, shoe manufacturers developed removable plastic "claws." When used in conjunction with replaceable variable length spikes, track shoes now have more versatility for different track surfaces. At this time, all major shoe manufacturers use a universal last, not a female last, for this shoe type.

Running Flats

A recent study of 60,000 high school athletes in the Seattle area shows that girls' cross-country running has the highest injury rate of any school sport, including football. One third of the female runners suffered an injury, with tendinitis of the knee, shin splints, ankle sprains, and stress fractures being the most common.[8] Many of these injuries were overuse injuries that could have been prevented with better conditioning and proper selection of running flats. More research and design has been done in the production of this shoe type than in all other areas of athletics footwear.

The features that are most required in a running shoe used for training on hard road surfaces are shock absorption, flexibility, control and stability in the heel counter area, torsional rigidity in the waist or shank, lightness, comfort, traction, motion control, and good fit (Fig. 34).

Because of the specific needs of individual runners, athletics shoe wear companies now produce models for specific foot types, gait patterns, and training styles. There are designs for light runners, heavy runners, heel strikers, lightweight trainers, and for motion control, stability, and rugged terrain. Many shoe companies are in the process of, or have developed, an anatomic female last for this shoe category. This segmentation of the market is crossing over into other major segments of the athletics shoe market, such as tennis and basketball.

Uppers usually are made of lightweight soft or mesh nylon. A rigid heel counter is necessary because most runners land heel first. The midsoles of training shoes should be lightweight and offer good cushioning properties. Although PU and EVA are the most commonly used midsole materials, ambient air, freon, and silicone gel can also be used. These materials are recommended for the female runner who may be suffering from stress fractures of the foot. All these materials have good to excellent shock absorbency and are built into heel wedge and midsole combinations. The shape of the sole is wedged from heel to toe. A flared heel increases stability in the heel area, a consideration for the female athlete who has suffered from inversion injuries at the ankle or from Achilles tendinitis.

Traction is obtained by rubber outsole materials and a good tread design. To obtain the best traction on loose or open terrain surfaces, a deeper sole tread is desired. On harder smooth surfaces, such as pavement, a lower profile tread offers good stability and adequate traction. Flexion path designs on the outsole at the metatarsophalangeal joints improve flexibility.

Walking Shoes

The walking shoe is one of the biggest and fastest growing categories of women's athletics shoes (Fig. 35). The design of this lightweight shoe is similar to that of a training running shoe and includes features needed in walking, such as a flexible forefoot; a comfortable, soft upper; and good shock absorption.

For the urban female walker, the weight of the shoe is not a very important consideration, and leather is often used for the upper material. An ample toe box and soft sock liner are added for comfort. The sole also is different from that of a standard running shoe in that a wedge is incorporated into the design. The tread has a smooth,

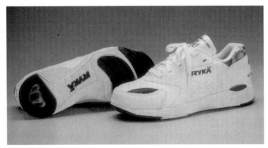

FIGURE 35
Walking shoe with a flexible forefoot, comfortable soft upper, good shock absorption, smooth tread, and rocker sole design. (Reproduced with permission from RYKÄ. Any illustrations of or statements about commercial products are solely the opinion(s) of the author(s) and do not represent an Academy endorsement or evaluation of these products.)

low profile with a herringbone pattern. Many outsoles have a rocker design to encourage the natural roll of the foot during the walking motion. This feature also helps reduce excessive flex at the metatarsophalangeal joints.

A walking shoe should have a firmer area on the heel for landing than most running shoes. The upswept heel of many running shoes does not offer the landing platform needed by walkers. Most walkers also benefit from the use of a more resilient material in the rear part of the shoe. A heel height of 10 to 15 mm is recommended for exercise walking to encourage the correct walking motion and reduce overstretching of the Achilles tendon, a risk in the female athlete.

COURT SPORT SHOES

Racquet Sports

Racquet sports require forward, backward, and side-to-side movements. The body must be moved with coordination and control in all directions. Court shoes used in racquet sports are subjected to heavy abuse, and wear patterns are produced in a short period of time. The female participant in racquet sports may suffer particularly from toenail and toe problems exacerbated by sudden stops, changes in direction, and jamming of the foot into the toe box.

Tennis

Tennis requires coordinated body moves with quick side-to side movement, sprinting, jumping, and stretching. The sport is played on lawn, clay, asphalt, synthetic, and rubberized courts. An appropriate sole must be made for each surface. On clay courts, soles with too deep a tread pattern may be prohibited because of excessive court wear even though most players would prefer the traction. On artificial or synthetic surfaces, harder soles with high rubber content or dual density PU are preferred for durability.

A tennis shoe should provide good lateral support, light to medium weight, a flat sole with a good heel wedge, a firm heel counter, a well-cushioned insole and midsole, good ventilation, an ample toe box, nonslip traction, a pivot point, and reinforcement for toe drag (Fig. 36). The upper should provide a high quarter pattern to give good ankle and lateral foot support. Over the ankle line, midcut models are available for those players who prefer additional ankle support.

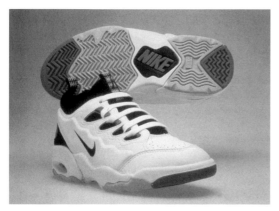

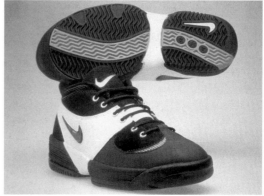

FIGURE 36

A tennis shoe should provide good lateral support, light to medium weight, a flat sole, a firm heel counter, a well-cushioned insole and midsole, an ample toe box, nonslip traction, a pivot point, and toe drag reinforcement. (Reproduced with permission from NIKE. Any illustrations of or statements about commercial products are solely the opinion(s) of the author(s) and do not represent an Academy endorsement or evaluation of these products.)

FIGURE 37

A basketball shoe should provide a flat sole, good lateral and medial support, light to medium weight, good cushioning, a large firm heel counter, toe drag reinforcement, ventilation, a pivot point, and good traction. (Reproduced with permission from NIKE. Any illustrations of or statements about commercial products are solely the opinion(s) of the author(s) and do not represent an Academy endorsement or evaluation of these products.)

Manufacturers of tennis shoes recommend more cushioning in the ball of the foot for the serve-and-volley player. For the baseline player, a firm heel counter, strong reinforcement in the heel and midfoot area, and good rear foot stability are recommended.

Basketball

The Athletic Footwear Association has noted that 41% of the basketball players younger than 17 years of age are female and that more high school girls play basketball than any other sport.[1] Basketball requires backward, forward, and vertical accelerations, quick stops, and side-to-side movements. The playing surface is usually wood but occasionally is synthetic or rubberized material. The basketball shoe should provide a flat sole, good lateral and medial support, light to medium weight, good cushioning, a slight heel wedge, a large firm heel counter, toe drag reinforcement, ventilation, a pivot point, and good traction (Fig. 37). A high rubber content in the sole is recommended. Soles with multiple-edge patterns, such as squares, circles, or diamonds, offer better traction than the herringbone design, which is excellent for forward stops but not for good lateral stops. High-cut designs are available for full ankle support but must not restrict ankle flexion. Proprioceptor straps are commonly used. Low-cut uppers are preferred by some players for better ankle flexibility, but the incidence of ankle injuries may increase with this type of shoe.[9]

The emphasis of recent design research in basketball shoes has been the prevention of inversion injuries to the ankle. Studies have shown that shoes with increasing amounts of ankle restriction in the upper significantly reduce ankle joint inversion.[10] However, it has also been shown that with increasing amounts of ankle restriction, movements are also restricted in the frontal plane, which leads to reduced agility. Therefore, a compromise in design must be met between performance and protection of the athlete. Because of increasing interest in this sport, most major shoe companies are introducing a line of women's basketball shoes.

SOCCER SHOES

An increasingly popular sport with women, soccer mainly involves kicking, running, jumping, sliding, stretching, and multidirectional movements. The playing surfaces are natural grass and artificial turf. Soccer is played almost entirely by the feet, with the ball being kicked off the medial, lateral, and dorsal aspects. Soccer shoe lasts tend to be snug fitting, often using narrow European lasts (Fig. 38). Soft and thinner leathers are preferred for the upper so players can feel the ball, but the

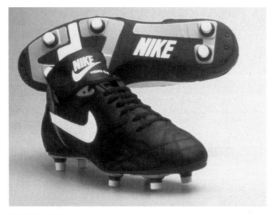

FIGURE 38
Soft and thinner leathers are preferred for the upper of most soccer shoes, because players like to feel the ball, but the tongue should be well padded to reduce lace pressure and protect the kicking area on the dorsum of the foot. (Reproduced with permission from NIKE. Any illustrations of or statements about commercial products are solely the opinion(s) of the author(s) and do not represent an Academy endorsement or evaluation of these products.)

tongue should be well padded to reduce lace pressure and protect the kicking area on the dorsum of the foot. Special lacing patterns may need to be used to accommodate the female with a high arch. Some players use the tongue and lace area to produce spin and control the ball. Soles should be flexible at the metatarsophalangeal joints for running and have torsional stability.

ICE SKATING BOOTS

The mechanics of skating are similar for all skating events, although footwear and blades are specialized for each event. Ankle movement and good support are necessary for skating performance. However, the subtalar joint must be free to allow positioning of the blade on the ice.

The traditional leather boot and the injection-molded model are the two main types of boots available. A leather boot should have good ankle support and a firm heel counter with elongation of the medial side. Uppers are made from thick grade leather or split leather with a leather or textile lining, which gives the foot and ankle stability but allows some flexibility. Metal eyelets are used in the lower portion of the throat, and metal hooks are used proximally.

ALPINE SKIING BOOTS

Alpine skiing requires ankle and knee flexion, forward lean, and balance on snow-covered surfaces. Ski boots provide a high-cut upper of a hinged or one piece injection-molded plastic outer shell to support the lower leg. The boot should provide rigid support for the foot and ankle and allow forward ankle flexion. Adjustable buckles, straps, or dial closure devices are used for instep support and a comfortable snug fit. More recently, buckles and overlaps on the vamp of rear- and midentry boots have been eliminated, reducing pressure on the instep and ankle regions. Inner liners can contain a footbed, a variety of wedges, or adjustable canting devices. To relieve pressure, conforming foam or pressure-flow bags can be used.

Ski boots are one of the last categories of athletics footwear to accommodate the female athlete. Many female skiers complain that their heels piston up and down, their ankles move side to side, and their instep is jammed up against the boot. The reason that many women's models fail to fit is that they only differ from men's models in cosmetics and the shape of the inner boot. The shell remains the same as in a men's boot. Boots are energy-transfer devices, and the foot cannot transfer energy unless it is in contact with the boot. If the shell is not close to the bones of the foot, the boot will not fit properly. Important design differences include an elevated heel for a shorter female Achilles tendon, easier forward flexion, and a more flared ankle cuff.

DANCING SHOES

Aerobic Dance

Aerobic dancing requires stationary skipping, running, jumping, stretching, dancing, and stair climbing. An aerobic dance shoe should be a combination of both a lightweight, shock-absorbent running shoe and a modified indoor court shoe (Fig. 39). Medial and lateral support is needed, as well as a wrap-up toe and heel protection. The forefoot requires stabilization and good shock absorption. EVA and PU combinations, air systems, and gel are used in shock-absorbing forefoot pads. Flexibility in the forepart is important.

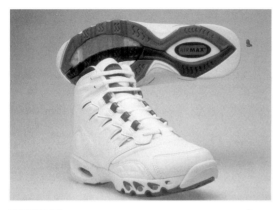

FIGURE 39
An aerobic shoe should be shock absorbent, provide medial and lateral support, a wrap-up toe, and heel protection. (Reproduced with permission from NIKE. Any illustrations of or statements about commercial products are solely the opinion(s) of the author(s) and do not represent an Academy endorsement or evaluation of these products.)

Ballet

Ballet slippers, like those used in gymnastics, are soft and come away from the midfoot when the foot is pointed. Pointe shoes tend to do the same though they are securely fixed to the heel. Ballerinas are unable to accommodate traditional orthotic devices in either their slippers or pointe shoes. However, orthoses can be devised. For patients who need arch support, a felt arch

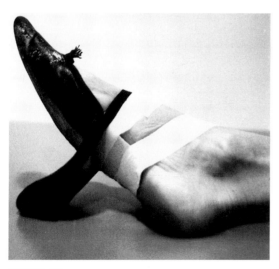

FIGURE 40
A soft ballet slipper with an orthosis taped to the dancer's foot.

support can be taped to the foot instead of being inserted in the shoe (Fig. 40). Ballerinas who must dance en pointe, but whose second toes are significantly shorter than their first, can equalize their toe lengths using either foam rubber toe caps, or a custom made molded toe box that fits inside the toe box of the pointe shoe.

REFERENCES

1. Pereira J: Women jump ahead of men in purchases of shoes. *Wall Street Journal,* May 26, 1995.

2. Hunter-Griffin LY (ed): Female athletes, in *Athletic Training and Sports Medicine,* ed 2. Rosemont, IL, American Academy of Orthopaedic Surgeons, 1991, pp 921-932.

3. Williams KR, Cavanaugh PR, Ziff JL: Biomechanical studies of elite female distance runners. *Int J Sports Med* 1987;8 (suppl 2): 107-118.

4. Valiant GA: The effect of outsole pattern on basketball shoe traction, in Terauds J, Gowitzke BA, Holt LE (eds): *Biomechanics in Sports III & IV:* Proceedings of the International Symposium of Biomechanics in Sports. Del Mar, CA, Research Center for Sports, 1987, pp 29-37.

5. Frey CC, Thompson F, Smith J, et al: American Orthopaedic Foot and Ankle Society women's shoe survey. *Foot Ankle* 1993;14:78-81.

6. Frey CC, Thompson F, Smith J: Update on women's footwear. *Foot Ankle* 1995;16:328-331.

7. Clarke TE, Frederick EC, Hamill CL: The effects of shoe design parameters on rear foot control in running. *Med Sci Sports Exerc* 1983; 15:376-381.

8. Bloom MS: Girls' cross-country taking a heavy toll, study shows. *New York Times,* December 4, 1993.

9. Garrick JG, Requa RK: Role of external support in the prevention of ankle sprains. *Med Sci Sports Exerc* 1973;5:200-203.

10. Robinson JR, Frederick EC, Cooper LB: Systematic ankle stabilization and the effect on performance. *Med Sci Sports Exerc* 1986;18:625-628.

THE FEMALE ATHLETE TRIAD

CAROL C. TEITZ, MD

The combination of disordered eating, amenorrhea, and osteoporosis is called the female athlete triad.[1] The factors in this triad are interdependent and can occur as a result of frequent and intense athletic participation.

DISORDERED EATING

Disordered eating ranges from a preoccupation with food and body image to severe problems, such as anorexia nervosa or bulimia. In athletes, depending on the sport studied, the prevalence of eating disorders ranges from 15% to 62%.[2,3] Some athletes try to control weight by excessive vigorous exercising. In a society that values "thinness," it is difficult to objectively examine nutritional habits and caloric intake. Nutritional problems are the greatest in women who participate in dance, and in sports, such as gymnastics, diving, and figure skating, in which body habitus is incorporated into subjective judging. These women sometimes starve themselves purposefully. Other times, they are subtly or overtly encouraged by their coaches and parents to strive for a body stereotypic for a specific sport. In the process of attempting to impose a universal but unrealistic standard of body shape, disordered eating may be encouraged. Athletes in sports with weight classifications, such as martial arts and rowing, also may be prone to eating disorders.

Women in other sports may have such high caloric demands that they don't take in sufficient numbers of calories to meet those demands. In endurance sports, excess body weight, especially in the form of fat, is often viewed by coaches and athletes as detrimental to performance. For performance, lean body mass is more important than percentage of body fat. Unfortunately, during extreme dieting, muscle mass is lost along with fat. This must be emphasized to the athlete. The problem is compounded when coaches and train-ers advise athletes on ideal body fat percentage using underwater weighing to measure body fat. The traditional formulae for calculating body composition by underwater weighing techniques rely on a standard value for bone density. In young women with amenorrhea and decreased bone density, these formulae will actually tend to overestimate the percentage of body fat.

Severe disturbances in eating behavior may be diagnosable as anorexia nervosa and bulimia (Outlines 3 and 4). These have in common an aberrant perception of body shape and weight. In the general population, 0.5% to 1% of adolescent and young adult women have anorexia nervosa, and 2% to 4% of adolescent and young adult women have bulimia.[4] Over 90% of athletes with anorexia or bulimia are adolescent girls and women.

Anorexia nervosa was first described in the late 19th century. Its current criteria include weight 15% below that expected for height and age, a morbid fear of fatness, abnormal body image, and amenorrhea.[4] Truly anorexic patients will be extremely thin and "bony" and may have fine downy baby hair (lanugo) on their bodies. Other findings may include cold intolerance, brittle hair and nails, bradycardia, constipation/bloating, and orthostatic hypotension. Elevated serum carotene can lead to a yellowish discoloration of hands and feet. Abnormal hematologic and electrolyte laboratory tests, and electrocardiograph findings may also be noted in advanced cases.[3]

Bulimia was first defined in 1976. Its criteria include binge eating two times per week for at least 3 months, purging, abnormal body image, and loss of control around eating. Bulimic women may have enlargement of the parotid glands (chipmunk cheeks), erosion of the enamel at the back of the teeth from recurrent vomiting of acidic stomach contents, and calluses on the back of the fingers from using them to induce vomiting (Russell's sign). Constipation, diarrhea, sore throat, chest pain, bloating, and abdominal

OUTLINE 3

DIAGNOSTIC CRITERIA FOR ANOREXIA NERVOSA

A. Refusal to maintain body weight at or above a minimally normal weight for age and height.

B. Intense fear of gaining weight or becoming fat, even though underweight.

C. Disturbance in the way in which one's body weight or shape is experienced, undue influence of body weight or shape on self-evaluation, or denial of the seriousness of the current low body weight.

D. In postmenarcheal females, amenorrhea, ie, the absence of at least three consecutive menstrual cycles.

(Adapted with permission from the American Psychiatric Association: *Diagnostic and Statistical Manual of Mental Disorders: DSM-IV*, ed 4. Washington, DC, American Psychiatric Association, 1994, pp 539-550.)

OUTLINE 4

DIAGNOSTIC CRITERIA FOR BULIMIA NERVOSA

A. Recurrent episodes of binge eating. An episode of binge eating is characterized by both of the following:

1. Eating, in a discrete period of time (eg, within any 2-hour period) an amount of food that is definitely larger than most people would eat during a similar period of time and under similar circumstances.

2. A sense of lack of control over eating during the episode (eg, a feeling that one cannot stop eating or control what or how much one is eating).

B. Recurrent inappropriate compensatory behavior in order to prevent weight gain, such as self-induced vomiting; misuse of laxatives, diuretics, enemas, or other medications; fasting; or excessive exercise.

C. The binge eating and inappropriate compensatory behaviors both occur, on average, at least twice a week for 3 months.

D. Self-evaluation is unduly influenced by body shape and weight.

E. The disturbance does not occur exclusively during episodes of anorexia nervosa.

(Adapted with permission from the American Psychiatric Association: *Diagnostic and Statistical Manual of Mental Disorders: DSM-IV*, ed 4. Washington, DC, American Psychiatric Association, 1994, pp 539-550.)

pain are common. In more advanced cases, orthostatic hypotension and abnormal laboratory values may be found.

Consequences of disordered eating range from impaired performance to death. Ten percent to 18% of women with untreated anorexia nervosa and bulimia may die from cardiac problems, blood chemical abnormalities, or suicide.[5-7] Insufficient caloric intake can result in decreased endurance, strength, speed, ability to concentrate, increased reaction time, and fluid and electrolyte imbalances. Problems with cardiovascular, gastrointestinal, and thermoregulatory systems also lead to a decrease in performance. In addition, insufficient caloric intake can also lead to menstrual disturbances and subsequent osteopenia.

ATHLETIC AMENORRHEA

Amenorrhea is present in up to 5% of the general population, excluding pregnant women, and in 10% to 20% of vigorously exercising women. Its prevalence may reach as high as 40% to 50% of elite runners and professional ballet dancers.[8-10] There is a complex interplay between the stress of intense training and normal ovulatory function.[11] Amenorrheic athletes are more likely to have

begun training at an earlier age than normally menstruating athletes. Although "athletic amenorrhea" was first thought to be caused by an insufficient amount of body fat,[12] it has subsequently been found to be a much more complex phenomenon. Whether athletic amenorrhea is an entity separate from that produced by weight loss or psychogenic cause is controversial. Body fat does play a role, although the stress of training and nutritional status are equally important. In athletes with insufficient caloric intake, the incidence of athletic amenorrhea rises regardless of percentage body fat.[13] Obviously athletes with low caloric intake may have low body fat. However, there are also athletes who have normal body fat but who consume less than the number of calories needed for intensive sports training. These women, too, become amenorrheic.

Amenorrhea can be classified as either primary or secondary. Primary amenorrhea is defined as no pubertal changes, such as breast buds, by 14 years of age, or no menstrual bleeding by the age of 16 years.[14] Secondary amenorrhea is defined as no menstrual cycles in a 6-month period in a woman who has had at least one episode of menstrual bleeding.[14] The onset of amenorrhea may be abrupt or gradual following an interval of oligomenorrhea (menstrual intervals greater than 35 days). The most common cause of amenorrhea is pregnancy. Amenorrhea also can be caused by structural abnormalities of the reproductive tract, testicular feminization, and hormonal abnormalities in the hypothalamic-pituitary-ovarian axis.[15] Athletic amenorrhea is thought to be a form of hypothalamic amenorrhea in which pulsatile gonadotropin releasing hormone (GnRH) is deficient, absent, or inappropriately secreted. In addition to tumors and congenital anomalies, psychological or physical stress can affect neurohormones that modulate GnRH. These include endogenous opioids, cortisol, melatonin, and dopamine. Increased levels of these neurohormones associated with endurance sports directly suppress the frequency and amplitude of GnRh pulses.[16-19] Lowered estrogen production by fat cells also results in abnormal feedback to the hypothalamus and resulting amenorrhea.

Some athletes have return of menses during intervals of rest even without weight gain or change in body fat. Resumption of normal menstrual cycles may take months or years after the stress is relieved. Prolonged amenorrhea can result in osteoporosis.[20,21]

OSTEOPOROSIS

Cann and associates[22] first described loss of bone mineral in the spines of young amenorrheic athletes in 1984. Since then, many authors have confirmed that amenorrhea induced by exercise results in bone mineral loss much like that seen after menopause.[23] Although high intensity exercise may increase bone mineral density at specific skeletal sites that are maximally stressed even in amenorrheic and oligomenorrheic athletes,[24-26] whole body bone mineral density is significantly lower in amenorrheic athletes than in controls.[22,27-30]

Osteoporosis may result from the failure to lay down a normal amount of bone during a critical time of life, from loss of bone that was already present, or from a combination of both. Sixty percent to 70% of a woman's peak bone mass is acquired before the age of 20 years. When the adolescent female athlete is amenorrheic and does not lay down a normal amount of bone during her adolescence, she may always have decreased bone mass.[31] Furthermore, this lost mineral cannot be restored by calcium or by hormone replacement.[32,33] Restoration of normal menses may retard the rate of further bone loss,[34] but the bone already lost is not replaced. Obviously, the implications for this group of women are frightening with regard to future risk of hip and spine fractures. Even in the present, the loss of bone is associated with an increased incidence of stress fractures.[35-37] Therefore, it is critical that the physician seeing the young female athlete with a stress fracture consider the possibility of early osteoporosis related to amenorrhea.

HISTORY AND PHYSICAL EXAMINATION

Screening questions should include menstrual history, nutritional history, and body weight history. While obtaining the menstrual history the physician should ask for the age of menarche, frequency and duration of menstrual periods, date of last menstrual period, and use of hormonal therapy. The nutritional history should include a 24-hour recall of food intake, the usual daily number of meals and snacks, and a list of forbidden foods (eg, meat or sweets). Body weight history should include the highest and lowest weights since menarche and the athlete's satisfaction with her present weight. What does she feel her ideal weight should be? Has she ever tried to control her weight using vomiting, laxatives, or diuretics?

ADDITIONAL STUDIES

In women with amenorrhea, it is important to rule out pregnancy and medical problems such as thyroid or pituitary disorders before ascribing amenorrhea solely to a woman's exercise program. Bone mineral density is most precisely measured indirectly by dual energy x-ray absorptiometry (DEXA). A typical DEXA scan submits the patient to less than 5 mrem per scan. This compares with a chest radiograph at 20 to 60 mrem or dental radiographs at 300 mrem.[38]

TREATMENT

Treatment of the female athlete triad requires a multidisciplinary approach, which includes physicians, a nutrition specialist, and often a psychologist or psychiatrist. For a high school or intercollegiate athlete, the physician should also involve the athletic trainer, the coach, and the patient's parents. The team physician is in the ideal position to screen for eating disorders and abnormal menses during the preparticipation physical examination. Furthermore, the orthopaedic surgeon seeing a young woman with a stress fracture should always consider the female athlete triad, particularly when a history of overuse is not forthcoming or when this is not the first stress fracture for this individual. The patient should be referred to a reproductive endocrinologist, gynecologist, or primary care physician familiar with the female athlete triad to check out the entire hypothalamic-pituitary-gonadal axis. If this workup is normal, chances are there is a nutritional factor or a stress-related factor, whether it be training stress or other life stresses, such as school work or family life. Treatment with replacement hormones may be necessary to prevent further bone loss.[39]

The patient should receive nutritional assessment and counseling from someone who understands athletics and caloric requirements. Disordered eating habits may be prevented with nutritional guidance and occasional estimation of an athlete's ideal weight range based on measurement of percent body fat using skinfold calipers or other methods. An adequate diet must include not only the appropriate caloric intake, but also at least 1,500 mg of calcium per day.[40] Treatment of more significant disordered eating may require contracts between physician and patient in which the level of sports participation is decreased or competition prohibited until the athlete reaches certain goals, such as a specific weight gain. The athlete may need psychological counseling as well, particularly if there is a true eating disorder, such as anorexia or bulimia, or for stress reduction techniques. Stress reduction techniques are particularly useful in the competitive athlete because they often help relieve performance anxiety. Additional educational materials about the female athlete triad can be obtained from the American College of Sports Medicine (ACSM) and the NCAA.

The combination of the female athlete triad and overuse frequently results in a high number of stress fractures, a particularly frustrating situation for a competitive athlete.

REFERENCES

1. Nattiv A, Yeager K, Drinkwater B, et al: The female athlete triad, in Agostini R, Titus S (eds): *Medical and Orthopedic Issues of Active and Athletic Women*. Philadelphia, PA, Hanley & Belfus, 1994, pp 169-174.

2. Rosen LW, McKeag DB, Hough DO, et al: Pathogenic weight-control behavior in female athletes. *Phys Sports Med* 1986;14:79-86.

3. Johnson MD: Disordered eating, in Agostini R, Titus S (eds): *Medical and Orthopedic Issues of Active and Athletic Women*. Philadelphia, PA, Hanley & Belfus, 1994, pp 141-151.

4. American Psychiatric Association: *Diagnostic and Statistical Manual of Mental Disorders: DSM-IV*, ed 4. Washington, DC, American Psychiatric Association, 1994, pp 539-550.

5. Palla B, Litt IF: Medical complications of eating disorders in adolescents. *Pediatrics* 1988; 81:613-623.

6. Pomeroy C, Mitchell JE: Medical issues in the eating disorders, in Brownell KD, Rodin J, Wilmore JH (eds): *Eating, Body Weight, and Performance in Athletes: Disorders of Modern Society*. Philadelphia, PA, Lea & Febiger, 1992, pp 202-221.

7. Kreipe RE, Harris JP: Myocardial impairment resulting from eating disorders. *Pediatr Ann* 1992;21:760-768.

8. Otis CL: Exercise-associated amenorrhea. *Clin Sports Med* 1992;11:351-362.

9. Marshall LA: Clinical evaluation of amenorrhea, in Agostini R, Titus S (eds): *Medical and Orthopedic Issues of Active and Athletic Women*. Philadelphia, PA, Hanley & Belfus, 1994, pp 152-163.

10. Warren MP: Clinical review 40: Amenorrhea in endurance runners. *J Clin Endocrinol Metab* 1992;75:1393-1397.

11. Loucks AB: Effects of exercise training on the menstrual cycle: Existence and mechanisms. *Med Sci Sports Exerc* 1990;22:275-280.

12. Frisch RE, McArthur JW: Menstrual cycles: Fatness as a determinant of minimum weight for height necessary for their maintenance or onset. *Science* 1974;185:949-951.

13. Baer JT, Taper LJ: Amenorrheic and eumenorrheic adolescent runners: Dietary intake and exercise training status. *J Am Diet Assoc* 1992;92:89-91.

14. Speroff L, Glass RH, Kase NG (eds): *Clinical Gynecologic Endocrinology and Infertility,* ed 4. Baltimore, MD, Williams & Wilkins, 1989, pp 165-211.

15. Loucks AB, Laughlin GA, Mortola JF, et al: Hypothalamic-pituitary-thyroidal function in eumenorrheic and amenorrheic athletes. *J Clin Endocrinol Metab* 1992;75:514-518.

16. De Cree C: Endogenous opioid peptides in the control of the normal menstrual cycle and their possible role in athletic menstrual irregularities. *Obstet Gynecol Surv* 1989;44:720-732.

17. Samuels MH, Sanborn CF, Hofeldt F, et al: The role of endogenous opiates in athletic amenorrhea. *Fertil Steril* 1991;55:507-512.

18. Laughlin GA, Loucks AB, Yen SS: Marked augmentation of nocturnal melatonin secretion in amenorrheic athletes, but not in cycling athletes: Unaltered by opioidergic or dopaminergic blockade. *J Clin Endocrinol Metab* 1991;73:1321-1326.

19. Hohtari H, Salimen-Lappalainen K, Laatikainen T: Response of plasma endorphins, corticotropin, cortisol, and luteinizing hormone in the corticotropin-releasing hormone stimulation test in eumenorrheic and amenorrheic athletes. *Fertil Steril* 1991;55:276-280.

20. Emans SJ, Grace E, Hoffer FA, et al: Estrogen deficiency in adolescents and young adults: Impact on bone mineral content and effects of estrogen replacement therapy. *Obstet Gynecol* 1990;76:585-592.

21. Voss L, Fadale P, Hulstyn M: Osteoporosis in young, athletic women. *J Musculoskel Med* 1996;13:15-22.

22. Cann CE, Martin MC, Genant HK, et al: Decreased spinal mineral content in amenorrheic women. *JAMA* 1984;251:626-629.

23. Myburgh KH, Bachrach LK, Lewis B, et al: Low bone mineral density at axial and appendicular sites in amenorrheic athletes. *Med Sci Sports Exerc* 1993;25:1197-1202.

24. Wolman RL, Clark P, McNally E, et al: Menstrual state and exercise as determinants of spinal trabecular bone density in female athletes. *Br Med J* 1990;301:516-518.

25. Snow-Harter C, Bouxsein ML, Lewis BT, et al: Effects of resistance and endurance exercise on bone mineral status of young women: A randomized exercise intervention trial. *J Bone Miner Res* 1992;7:761-769.

26. Slemenda CW, Johnston CC: High intensity activities in young women: Site specific bone mass effects among female figure skaters. *Bone Miner* 1993;20:125-132.

27. Drinkwater BL, Nilson K, Chesnut CH III, et al: Bone mineral content of amenorrheic and eumenorrheic athletes. *N Engl J Med* 1984; 311:277-281.

28. Lindberg JS, Fears WB, Hunt MM, et al: Exercise-induced amenorrhea and bone density. *Ann Intern Med* 1984;101:647-648.

29. Linnell SL, Stager JM, Blue PW, et al: Bone mineral content and menstrual regularity in female runners. *Med Sci Sports Exerc* 1984;16:343-348.

30. Marcus R, Cann C, Madvig P, et al: Menstrual function and bone mass in elite women distance runners: Endocrine and metabolic features. *Ann Intern Med* 1985;102:158-163.

31. Jonnavithula S, Warren MP, Fox RP, et al: Bone density is compromised in amenorrheic women despite return of menses: A 2-year study. *Obstet Gynecol* 1993;81:669-674.

32. Drinkwater BL, Chesnut CH III: Abstract: Site specific skeletal response to increased calcium in amenorrheic athletes. *Med Sci Sports Exerc* 1992;24:S45.

33. Weltman A, Snead DB, Weltman JY, et al: Abstract: Effects of calcium supplementation on bone mineral density (BMD) in premenopausal women runners. *Med Sci Sports Exerc* 1992; 24:S12.

34. Drinkwater BL, Nilson K, Ott S, et al: Bone mineral density after resumption of menses in amenorrheic athletes. *JAMA* 1986;256:380-382.

35. Barrow GW, Saha S: Menstrual irregularity and stress fractures in collegiate female distance runners. *Am J Sports Med* 1988;16:209-216.

36. Myburgh KH, Hutchins J, Fataar AB, et al: Low bone density is an etiologic factor for stress fractures in athletes. *Ann Intern Med* 1990;113:754-759.

37. Kadel NJ, Teitz CC, Kronmal RA: Stress fractures in ballet dancers. *Am J Sports Med* 1992;20:445-449.

38. Johnston CC Jr, Melton LJ III: Bone density measurement and the management of osteoporosis, in Favus MJ (ed): *Primer on the Metabolic Bone Diseases and Disorders of Mineral Metabolism,* ed 2. New York, NY, Raven Press, 1993, pp 136-146.

39. Haenggi W, Casez J, Birkhaeuser M, et al: Bone mineral density in young women with long-standing amenorrhea: Limited effect of hormone replacement therapy with ethinyl-estradiol and desogestrel. *Osteoporos Int* 1994;4:99-103.

40. Position of the American Dietetic Association and the Canadian Dietetic Association: Nutrition for physical fitness and athletic performance for adults. *J Am Diet Assoc* 1993;93:691-696.

STRESS FRACTURES

CAROL C. TEITZ, MD

Stress fractures, also known as fatigue fractures, were first described in the military, where they were known as march fractures. These fractures occurred when unconditioned recruits were subjected to strenuous activity. Bone is capable of adapting to increasing loads when the rate of increase is gradual. However, when even relatively normal loads are applied so frequently that the usual adaptive processes cannot occur, stress fracture results.[1]

When the stress loading frequency is optimal, bone formation and resorption are balanced. However, these adaptive phenomena will occur only in a normal hormonal milieu. Although exercise stimulates bone formation, exercise also produces systemic and circulatory changes that may affect bone homeostasis. Mild exercise appears to maintain bone but does not increase it. Higher resistance activities increase bone mass, diameter, and strength.[2] On the other hand, extensive exercise can produce relative caloric deficiency and hormonal imbalances that result in amenorrhea. Amenorrhea leads to bone mineral loss, which resembles postmenopausal osteoporosis. The hormonal influence in this setting seems to have a more potent effect on the bone than the influence of the physical stresses produced by the exercise.[3-8] Therefore, although recognized causes of stress fracture include poor training, equipment, environmental factors, and variations in anatomic alignment, fractures occurring as a result of decreased bone mineral density are of particular concern in the young female athlete.[9-11]

HISTORY AND PHYSICAL EXAMINATION

The clinical diagnosis of stress fracture is based on a history of the insidious onset of pain with percussive loading of the lower extremity. Although the patient may be able to walk without pain, typically she cannot run, jump, or dance.

Often there is a history of overuse, a change in shoewear or exercise surface, and the physical finding of tenderness to palpation of a discrete area of bone. Occasionally, when a stress fracture is present in the foot, it will appear swollen and red and make the physician think of an inflammatory or infectious process. When the symptoms are in the leg, the physician must consider periostitis, tendinitis, and chronic compartment syndrome. In either site, the differential diagnosis must include complete fracture, osteomyelitis, osteoid osteoma, or other tumor. Stress fractures in the the female that deserve special comment occur in the pubic ramus and in the ribs.

PUBIC RAMUS

Pubic ramus stress fractures present similarly in men and women, ie, with groin pain and tenderness to palpation of the ramus. However, to prevent recurrence, the physician should consider two etiologic factors that occur more commonly in women. One is a cross-over running style (Fig. 41), and the other is overstriding. The term "cross-over running" connotes excessive adduction of the lower extremity across the line of gait progression. This style may occur more commonly in women because of their wider pelves. Overstriding connotes excessive flexion of the lower extremity either to gain speed or to keep up with a taller running partner. Both cross-over running and overstriding create chronic pull by the adductor musculature at its origin on the pubic ramus. Sometimes this pull results in adductor tendinitis; other times it results in pubic ramus stress fractures. Information about running habits should be sought during the history so that, once the fracture heals, the patient is not returned to the identical environment in which the fracture occurred.

RIBS

Female rowers and golfers are particularly prone to stress fractures of the ribs, which are thought

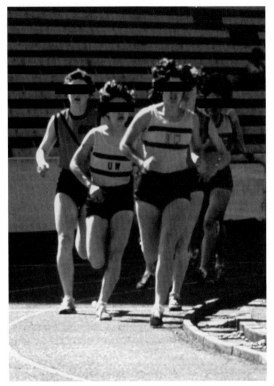

FIGURE 41
A cross-over running style, such that one foot lands directly in front of the other, can produce excessive strain in the adductor muscles and indirectly on their pubic origins.

to be caused by bending stresses applied to the posterolateral rib during repetitive pull by the serratus anterior, rhomboids, and trapezius muscles.[12] In rowers, these stress fractures are more common in scullers than sweepers.

The patient presents with posterolateral chest pain, which may be periscapular or may radiate around the rib anteriorly. The pain will be aggravated by rowing or by rotation of the torso during golf. When the fracture is complete, pain will be exacerbated by deep breathing and coughing. A patient's sleeping on her side may also produce pain. The involved rib will be tender to palpation, and pain may be increased by either anteroposterior or lateral compression of the rib cage. Radiographs may be negative, but bone scan will be positive. The patient may obtain relief by refraining from exacerbating activities, wearing a rib belt, and sleeping on her back. Once the fracture is nontender, special emphasis should be placed on serratus anterior and rhomboid strengthening. The rower should return to sweeping before she returns to sculling.

ADDITIONAL STUDIES

A stress fracture usually takes the form of a crack through the bone with no displacement. In many cases, the crack is not visible on routine radiographs. If movement at the fracture site is minimal, radiographically evident callus may not form. In other cases, the stress fracture can be recognized radiographically during the resorption phase between 7 and 10 days following fracture (Fig. 42, *left*). Callus formation is most commonly seen in metatarsal stress fractures, and thickening of the cortex is seen in tibial stress fractures.

Technetium diphosphonate bone scans (Fig. 42, *right*) are useful diagnostically when stress fractures are invisible on routine radiographs. When trying to distinguish stress fractures in the tibia from shin splints (periostitis), the physician should obtain both a scan in the "blood pool phase" and a delayed scan. Recent stress fractures are positive in the blood pool phase, whereas periostitis is not.[13] In addition, the physician should look at the actual scan and not just the report. Some radiologists will not diagnose a stress fracture unless the increased isotopic uptake crosses the entire diameter of the bone. In fact, many stress fractures are unicortical and may show increased uptake only in one cortex. The pattern of uptake is more helpful in distinguishing stress fracture from periostitis. Stress fractures are typically discrete areas of increased uptake whose longitudinal dimensions do not exceed 20% of the length of the bone. In contrast, periostitis typically extends along one cortex for lengths up to 30% to 75% of the length of the bone. As a result of continued remodeling at the fracture site, bone scans often remain "hot" for up to a year after the time of fracture and are not useful for assessing fracture healing. Bone scans need not be ordered routinely.

Computed tomography is useful in delineating stress fracture of the tarsal navicular and in distinguishing stress fracture from osteoid osteoma when radiographs reveal sclerosis with a central lucency.[14]

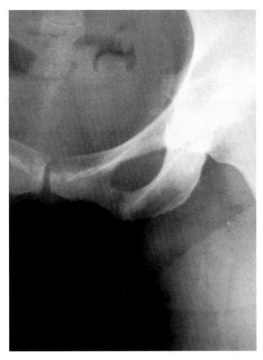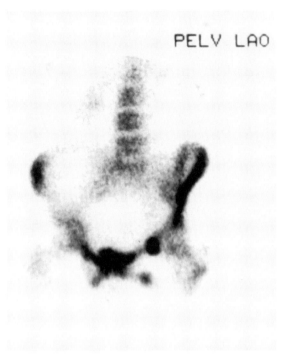

FIGURE 42
Left, A stress fracture is visible in the inferior pubic ramus. **Right,** The bone scan reveals the stress fracture seen on the radiograph (left) as well as an additional fracture in the superior pubic ramus.

Magnetic resonance images (MRI) are especially useful when trying to differentiate tumors, such as osteoid osteoma, from stress fractures, and in the pediatric setting where physeal isotopic uptake on bone scan sometimes makes visualization of stress fractures difficult.[15] MRI will reveal intramedullary bands of low signal intensity that are continuous with the cortex (the fracture) as well as intramedullary areas of high signal intensity on STIR images (the edema).[16] MRI has also shown a stress fracture in a case in which the bone scan was negative.[17]

If the clinical picture is typical for stress fracture and the radiograph is negative, the physician can treat the patient empirically. On the other hand, if the patient does not want to refrain from impact activities or wants to participate in an imminent athletic competition and there is concern about the risk of frank fracture, the physician should proceed with other imaging modalities to prove to the patient that a fracture is indeed present and the limb should be rested.

TREATMENT

During treatment of a lower extremity stress fracture, significant impact must be avoided, but other uses of the limb will provide the stresses necessary for growth of normal collagenous and skeletal tissue. For example, in a runner with a lower extremity stress fracture, running should be prohibited, but walking, swimming, rowing, and bicycling are suggested as alternative means of remaining fit, using the limbs, and avoiding further injurious forces. The limits and the activities allowed are a function of the location of the fracture. Crutches are prescribed when the patient cannot bear weight without discomfort and are used until the patient can walk without pain.

Immobilization is used for stress fractures in the leg or foot when there is concern about compliance or when the patient cannot tolerate crutches. For tibial or fibular stress fractures, pneumatic splints or removable "walkers" made of soft material and reinforced with plastic side pieces can be used to immobilize the fracture, obviate the need for crutches, and avoid "cast disease." The pneumatic splints can be obtained in varying lengths and sometimes allow earlier return to activity for patients with tibial stress fractures.[18,19] Neither pneumatic splints nor removable walkers are suitable forms of immobilization for stress fractures in the foot. Internal fixation may be required for certain stress fractures in the femoral neck,[20] the anterior tibial cortex,[21] and the tarsal navicular.[22]

Nonsteroidal anti-inflammatory drugs (NSAIDs) are contraindicated in the treatment of pain related to stress fractures. There is evidence that suggests NSAIDs will interfere with fracture healing.[23] Although this interference has not been specifically demonstrated, NSAIDs are used successfully to decrease the incidence of heterotopic ossification after total joint replacement[24] and after muscle trauma.[25] Therefore, it is possible to infer that they potentially could interfere with new bone formation after a fracture. When chemical methods of pain control are needed, acetaminophen usually suffices.

The fracture is healed when it is no longer tender to palpation, and the patient is able to tolerate impact.[26] Progressive return to the desired activity levels ensues. When the patient can walk without discomfort, she can begin an "amphibious" rehabilitation program. The patient begins by jogging in water that is chest high and gradually moves up to waist-high water. Then she moves out of the water and onto the land. The decrease in buoyancy provides a gradually increasing load to the bone, giving it a chance to adapt. The next step is sport-specific rehabilitation, which starts with a time or distance that is about a third of where the patient was at the time of fracture. For example, if the patient suffered a stress fracture while running 30 miles per week, she should start at 10 miles per week, divided into three runs of just over 3 miles each. These are run on alternate days, with a 2-day rest. The mileage is then increased at 10% to 15% per week.[27] Similarly, someone who was participating in a dance class 3 days per week should try one class per week for 1 month and then add one class per week each subsequent month. If the type of dance involves jumping, that part of the class should be omitted initially and gradually introduced.

Included in this rehabilitation must be modification of contributing factors that may have been identified. One of the elements of overuse injuries that distinguishes them from other musculoskeletal injuries is that the victim of an overuse injury is routinely returned to "the scene of the crime." In other words, after treating the injury, the physician sends the patient back into the situation in which she was injured. Therefore, to avoid recurrence, it is critical to identify any correctable factors that contributed to the injury.

First is the training schedule. Modifications include training different body parts on different days, alternating days, or varying the frequency, intensity, and duration of training. These modifications allow the musculoskeletal tissues a chance to adapt. Second, if a biomechanical factor was identified, either in the patient's sports equipment or anatomic structure, this factor should be changed where possible. Arch supports can be provided; shock absorption can be increased either in an orthosis, shoe, or the surface on which the person will be exercising. Metatarsal bars, pads, or Morton's extension orthoses can be obtained. Proper shoes for the sport should be purchased, and shoes should be in good condition. The typical shock absorbency of running shoes is about 600 miles. If a worn-out shoe was a contributing factor, all that may be needed is a new shoe. Third, if abnormal menses are present, attention should be drawn to this, particularly if the patient has had more than one stress fracture.

REFERENCES

1. Chamay A, Tschantz P: Mechanical influences in bone remodeling: Experimental research on Wolff's law. *J Biomech* 1972;5:173-180.

2. Dalen N, Olsson KE: Bone mineral content and physical activity. *Acta Orthop Scand* 1974;45:170-174.

3. Cann CE, Martin MC, Genant HK, et al: Decreased spinal mineral content in amenorrheic women. *JAMA* 1984;251:626-629.

4. Drinkwater BL, Nilson K, Chesnut CH III, et al: Bone mineral content of amenorrheic and eumenorrheic athletes. *N Engl J Med* 1984; 311:277-281.

5. Lindberg JS, Fears WB, Hunt MM, et al: Exercise-induced amenorrhea and bone density. *Ann Intern Med* 1984;101:647-648.

6. Linnell SL, Stager JM, Blue PW, et al: Bone mineral content and menstrual regularity in female runners. *Med Sci Sports Exerc* 1984;16:343-348.

7. Marcus R, Cann C, Madvig P, et al: Menstrual function and bone mass in elite women distance runners: Endocrine and metabolic features. *Ann Intern Med* 1985;102:158-163.

8. Drinkwater BL, Bruemner B, Chesnut CH III: Menstrual history as a determinant of current bone density in young athletes. *JAMA* 1990;263:545-548.

9. Barrow GW, Saha S: Menstrual irregularity and stress fractures in collegiate female distance runners. *Am J Sports Med* 1988;16:209-216.

10. Myburgh KH, Hutchins J, Fataar AB, et al: Low bone density is an etiologic factor for stress fractures in athletes. *Ann Intern Med* 1990;113:754-759.

11. Kadel NJ, Teitz CC, Kronmal RA: Stress fractures in ballet dancers. *Am J Sports Med* 1992;20:445-449.

12. Holden DL, Jackson DW: Stress fractures of the ribs in female rowers. *Am J Sports Med* 1985;13:342-348.

13. Rupani HD, Holder LE, Espinola DA, et al: Three-phase radionuclide bone imaging in sports medicine. *Radiology* 1985;156:187-196.

14. Murcia M, Brennan RE, Edeiken J: Computed tomography of stress fracture. *Skeletal Radiol* 1982;8:193-195.

15. Horev G, Korenreich L, Ziv N, et al: The enigma of stress fractures in the pediatric age: Clarification or confusion through the new imaging modalities. *Pediatr Radiol* 1990;20:469-471.

16. Tyrrell PN, Davies AM: Magnetic resonance imaging appearances of fatigue fractures of the long bones of the lower limb. *Br J Radiol* 1994;67:332-338.

17. Pistolesi GF, Caudana R, D'Attoma N, et al: Case report 686: Stress fracture at the distal end of femur simulating "periosteal desmoid". *Skeletal Radiol* 1991;20:454-457.

18. Dickson TB Jr, Kichline PD: Functional management of stress fractures in female athletes using a pneumatic leg brace. *Am J Sports Med* 1987;15:86-89.

19. Whitelaw GP, Wetzler MJ, Levy AS, et al: A pneumatic leg brace for the treatment of tibial stress fractures. *Clin Orthop* 1991;270:301-305.

20. Devas MB: Stress fractures of the femoral neck. *J Bone Joint Surg* 1965;47B:728-738.

21. Beals RK, Cook RD: Stress fractures of the anterior tibial diaphysis. *Orthopedics* 1991;14:869-875.

22. Torg JS, Pavlov H, Cooley LH, et al: Stress fractures of the tarsal navicular: A retrospective review of twenty-one cases. *J Bone Joint Surg* 1982;64A:700-712.

23. DiCesare PE, Nimni ME, Peng L, et al: Effects of indomethacin on demineralized bone-induced heterotopic ossification in the rat. *J Orthop Res* 1991;9:855-861.

24. Kjaersgaard-Anderson P, Nafei A, Teichert G, et al: Indomethacin for prevention of heterotopic ossification: A randomized controlled study in 41 hip arthroplasties. *Acta Orthop Scand* 1993;64:639-642.

25. Garland DE: A clinical perspective on common forms of acquired heterotopic ossification. *Clin Orthop* 1991;263:13-29.

26. Taunton JE, Clement DB, Webber D: Lower extremity stress fractures in athletes. *Phys Sportsmed* 1981;9:77-86.

27. Teitz CC: Overuse injuries, in Teitz CC (ed): *Scientific Foundations of Sports Medicine.* Toronto, Canada, BC Decker, 1989, pp 299-328.

SPECIAL PROBLEMS

CAROL C. TEITZ, MD

SPECIAL POPULATIONS

THE "OLDER ATHLETE"

With the current emphasis on the health benefits of regular exercise, more women are beginning exercise programs in the perimenopausal and postmenopausal age groups. Other women, who have been exercising for years, may find as they get older, that their knees, feet, or backs are beginning to hurt. Both groups may present requesting advice on safe, painless, and beneficial exercise programs.

First, as always, the physician should obtain a complete medical history so that previous medical and musculoskeletal problems can be addressed. When there are cardiac or pulmonary considerations, consultation with the patient's primary-care physician is appropriate before suggesting specific forms of exercise. Patients with significant anatomic problems in the lower extremity, such as markedly pronated feet, marked genu valgum, or extreme femoral anteversion, that cannot be compensated for with orthoses or muscle strengthening should be steered away from weightbearing exercise. They can be encouraged to participate in aquaerobics, bicycling, swimming, and sometimes rowing. On the other hand, patients with chronic shoulder problems will do better avoiding swimming or using their arms during aerobic dance classes. If they are interested in weight lifting, patients with shoulder pain also should be advised to avoid overhead use of their arms and to keep their arms below the horizontal level of their shoulders while exercising. Patients with lower extremity arthritis should avoid lower extremity activities involving a lot of impact, such as running, volleyball, or aerobic dance. However, many of these patients will be able to tolerate limited impact sports such as tennis, especially if they wear shoes with good shock absorption or add shock-absorbing insoles to their shoes.

Women with osteoporosis need to be more careful about lifting weights. If they wish to work out with weights, they should be encouraged to use light weights and work toward increasing repetitions. Proper breathing during exercise to avoid Valsalva's maneuvers is also important.

When structured vigorous athletic activities are not compatible with the physical status of the patient, caloric expenditure can be increased by encouraging patients to take stairs instead of elevators, walking or cycling to the store instead of driving, or engaging in yard and house work. When the senior athlete presents with limb pain, the orthopaedist must remember the increased likelihood in this age group of cancer, both primary and metastatic, as a cause for local or referred pain.

EXERCISE DURING PREGNANCY

Musculoskeletal problems in the physically active pregnant woman are related to weight gain, ligamentous relaxation, lordosis, and change in the center of gravity. Near term, running sports become more difficult as the weight and bulk of the abdomen increase. In the third trimester, exercise in water is advocated because the buoyant effect reduces the stress of weightbearing. There is concern that impact sports or sports requiring a lot of torque may cause membrane rupture, placental separation, umbilical cord entanglement, or direct fetal injury. The absolute intensity of weightbearing exercise also should decrease as pregnancy progresses because the oxygen demands during weightbearing exercise increase during pregnancy. It is difficult to judge the intensity of maternal exercise using the usual criterion of heart rate because pregnancy increases maternal blood volume, heart rate, and cardiac output.

Researching the effects of exercise in pregnancy is difficult because of the great variety of types of exercise, exercise intensities, and durations that may have very different maternal and fetal effects. There is contradictory evidence concerning the influence of exercise on the onset of labor, course of labor, and fetal growth. Nevertheless, most physically fit women with normal pregnancies may continue their regular program of exercise without having an adverse effect on most aspects of labor and fetal growth.

Many of the concerns related to exercise during pregnancy focus on the safety of the fetus rather than problems occurring in the athlete herself. The concerns center principally around fetal hyperthermia and the risk of neural tube defects, insufficient placental blood flow, and adequate glucose availability for the fetus.[1]

Temperature elevation is proportional to exercise intensity. A well-conditioned athlete can dissipate heat through sweating; however, a poorly trained athlete is more likely to become hyperthermic. Dehydration and hot, humid environmental conditions will increase the likelihood of raised body temperature during exercise. Intense training can raise rectal temperature above the level found to be teratogenic in sheep (39.2° C). No prospective studies have demonstrated temperature elevation to be a teratogen in humans.

Although plasma volume expansion occurs as a result of both exercise and pregnancy and may help maintain uterine blood flow, prolonged exercise also decreases splanchnic blood flow to 40% to 50% of resting levels. Because the uterine circulation is part of the splanchnic bed, there are concerns, again based on observations in sheep, about decreased blood flow to the placenta during exercise. Glucose is a major fetal fuel and its availability is a function of glucose levels in maternal blood. Glucose utilization by the muscles during exercise will decrease levels of circulating glucose and may limit fetal glucose availability.

History and Physical Examination

One of the most common complaints in the pregnant woman, particularly in the second or third trimester, is that of back pain. It may or may not have a radicular component and is normally aggravated by activities in the standing position. Sensory, motor, or deep tendon reflexes changes are rarely present. Most commonly a Patrick's test will produce pain consistent with strain in the sacroiliac ligaments (see "Sacroiliac Pain", p.32).

Treatment

Back pain can be decreased by switching from standing activities, such as running or dancing, to sitting activities, such as rowing or bicycling. Abdominal support straps may provide symptomatic relief as will pelvic tilts and "angry cat" exercises (producing lumbar kyphosis) while face down on hands and knees.

Recommendations for exercise during pregnancy are found in Outline 5.[2] In summary, the pregnant athlete should try to maintain core body temperature less than 38°C. Diabetes, hypertension, history of miscarriage, multiple gestation, or

OUTLINE 5

ABRIDGED ACOG RECOMMENDATIONS FOR EXERCISE DURING PREGNANCY

1. Regular exercise (at least three times per week) is preferable to intermittent activity.

2. Women should avoid exercise in the supine position after the first trimester.

3. Pregnant women should stop exercising when fatigued and not exercise to exhaustion.

4. Exercise in which loss of balance could be detrimental to maternal or fetal well-being is contraindicated. Further, any type of exercise involving the potential for even mild abdominal trauma should be avoided.

5. Pregnancy requires an additional 300 kcal/d in order to maintain metabolic homeostasis. Women who exercise during pregnancy should be particularly careful to ensure an adequate diet.

6. Pregnant women who exercise in the first trimester should augment heat dissipation by ensuring adequate hydration, appropriate clothing, and optimal environmental surroundings during exercise.

7. Many of the physiologic and morphologic changes of pregnancy persist 4 to 6 weeks postpartum. Prepregnancy exercise routines should be resumed gradually.

(Reproduced with permission from the American College of Obstetrics and Gynecology: Exercise during pregnancy and the postpartum period. Technical Bulletin No. 189, Feb 1994.)

cervical defects are contraindications to exercise during pregnancy. The pregnant athlete may need to omit contact sports and diving from her exercise choices. Vigorous exercise programs should not be undertaken by unfit women during pregnancy, especially during the first trimester. The type of exercises recommended should minimize the risk of injury, while including the patient's preferences, and it should be coordinated with the physician managing the patient's pregnancy.

REHABILITATION AND EXERCISE PRESCRIPTION

In general, female athletes respond to rehabilitation in the same way as male athletes.[3] However, there are some technical points that are worth noting. First of all, most women except for those who have gone through college since Title IX,[4] have had little or no exposure to weight rooms and training techniques. Although many know about proper stretching methods, warm-up, and cool down, they may need to be educated about training principles such as specificity of training, muscle overload, and concentric and eccentric exercise (positive and negative work). Women may need someone in the weight room to explain and demonstrate proper use, and to act as a spotter as they begin using weights and strengthening machines.

Second, many of the machines in weight rooms are not configured for women. Particularly for small women, the lever arms may be too long or the lowest weight setting may be too heavy. Women may need to begin weight work with rubber tubing or free weights. Not only are light weights less likely to lead to injury, but they provide the opportunity to learn proper technique.

Third, because women in general tend to be weaker in their upper extremities, load increases for shoulder, chest, and arm exercises for women should probably be in the range of 2.5 to 5 lb rather than the typical 10-lb increases used for males and for the lower extremities.[5]

Fourth, some women are concerned about walking into a weight room and with how they look. These women will do better with individual, personalized instruction. Women tend to berate their own performance in activities that are not traditionally "feminine." Women who are not used to participating in athletics do better when they are not competing with others and when they are provided with immediate, objective, and accurate feedback.[6]

Fifth, motivational factors are somewhat different in men than in women. Although both sexes are motivated to exercise by a desire for fitness and good health, men also are influenced by enjoyment of competition and desire for physical excellence whereas some women are more likely than men also to be motivated by appearance and by opportunities for socialization.[7] These women are more likely to adhere to an exercise program if it is a group or partnered activity.

Finally, women, influenced by the media, have a tendency to work isolated muscle groups, often in an attempt to "spot reduce" or tone. They need to be taught that all muscles must be strengthened in order to most effectively transfer force from one body part to another. At least one exercise should be included for all large muscle groups, such as shoulder, back, chest, arms, abdomen, hips, thighs, and calves. Circuit training often accomplishes these goals.

When advising women on an exercise program, in addition to considering level of fitness and athletic interests, the exercise plan should be based on the patient's long-term goals. Progress toward these long-term goals can be made by replacing them with reasonable short-term goals. These goals should be sufficiently challenging, but not unreachable, so that positive reinforcement is readily achieved.

Identify potential obstacles to an exercise program such as child care, weather, or financial ability to join a gym. Encourage the patient to keep track of her exercise sessions and to reward herself for completing each session. Ultimately, the activity itself becomes the reward. Sometimes behavioral contracts are necessary between physician and patient. Also, make sure that the patient has proper clothing and equipment to prevent injury.[8]

PSYCHOSOCIAL ISSUES

ROLE MODELS

With the exception of the Olympics, female athletes are still rarely seen in the media, perhaps because of the lack of professional sports opportunities for women. Therefore, there is still a paucity of female athletic role models. Successful athletes are often competitive, physically strong, and achievement oriented. Female athletes also tend to be more intrinsically motivated, independent, and self-sufficient than nonathletic women. These traits are still considered by some to be masculine. How these traits are perceived by an individual girl are a function of her family, community, and culture.[9] Girls tend to drop out of athletics most often during their teens when peer pressure to appear "feminine" may be at its highest. Adults can help by trying to provide positive role models and pointing out that the personality characterstics noted above are also potentially useful in the workplace. A positive sports experience also carries over to increase self esteem.

THE "HAS BEEN"

For a young athlete who is unable to continue at the same level of participation or competition because of body changes brought on by puberty, the psychological impact can be devastating. This situation is common in gymnasts, dancers, and skaters, who may have spent all their "free" time training. Some of these adolescent girls, whose lives have centered around sports, will move on successfully to a different level of participation or a different sport altogether. Others may refocus on socialization, academic, or occupational goals. Still others may need professional counseling, particularly when their parents were also highly invested, both emotionally and financially, in what might have been a future as an elite athlete or professional dancer.[10]

For the mature athlete with body changes brought on by aging, many of the same issues exist. These women should be encouraged to try a different sport more attuned to their current physical abilities (see "Special Populations").

DISPROPORTIONAL PAIN SYNDROMES

Reflex sympathetic dystrophy, also called reflex neurovascular dystrophy (RND), is three times more prevalent in the female than in the male, particularly in adolescents. The term RND is preferable because it removes the potential misunderstanding on the part of the patient and family, that there is "sympathy" involved.[11] It also reflects the physiologic relationship of the nerves and cutaneous blood vessels. Sherry and associates[12,13]

described an additional clinical presentation similar to RND in childhood, but without the physical findings of aberrant sympathetic tone. These clinical syndromes probably represent a spectrum of the same physiologic process with the differences being largely semantic. The diagnosis of RND should always be kept in the back of the physician's mind when evaluating a teenage female athlete, especially when the information obtained during history and physical examination does not quite add up.

RND is typically the patient's subconscious way of dealing with an untenable situation either in her family, at school, or between her abilities and self-expectations.[14] Sherry (DD Sherry, MD, Children's Hospital and Medical Center, Seattle, WA, 1996, personal communication) suggests that girls take out stress on their own bodies, whereas boys take out stress on other people's bodies. The resulting psychosomatic pain syndrome relieves stress by focusing attention onto the patient, reducing expectations of achievement, or interrupting family conflict.[5] RND often begins with a minor musculoskeletal injury that appropriately induces some sympathetic response of discomfort, vasodilatation, and possible swelling. Unfortunately, because of the networking of the sympathetic nervous system with centers of emotion in the brain, in some patients the sympathetic nerves begin to function erratically, producing either too much sympathetic output or not enough.

History and Physical Examination

Most physicians are familiar with shoulder-hand syndrome, a form of RND that occurs in the post-traumatic setting. However, in the adolescent female, RND usually is insidious in onset and can appear to be infection or arthritis. The psychosomatic type may lack the autonomic physical findings associated with RND. Adolescents with RND and those with psychosomatic musculoskeletal pain have similar demographics, pain, disability, and psychodynamics and respond similarly to treatment. They differ in that the psychosomatic patients more frequently have less hyperesthesia and have intermittent pain that is more likely to be present at multiple or bilateral sites.[13]

The patient typically presents with a painful limb or joint and with significant disability related to the pain. The disability is the outstanding characteristic and markedly shadows the physical findings if any are present. Most patients have limited their activities. Symptoms are often exacerbated by stress, and the patient should be asked if she has noted this association. The pain is described as continuous in 63% of patients,[13] and lower extremity complaints predominate. In addition, the patients with psychosomatic musculoskeletal pain are usually high achievers either in sports, in academics, or both, who tend to deny negative feelings and try instead to please others. Depression is uncommon. There often are psychosocial problems in the patient herself or within her family. Two predominant types of abnormal family milieu commonly are seen: one is cohesive, stable, and organized, but intolerant of separation and individuation; the other is chaotic and emotionally unsupportive, with high levels of conflict.[13]

During the physical examination, an incongruent effect has been found in 96% of the psychosomatic patients, such that the patient is describing excruciating pain with a smile on her face. Frequently there is abnormal enmeshment with the parent if he or she is present in the examination room. The patient may not make eye contact with the examiner and questions directed at the patient may be answered by the parent. The involved limb may be red, swollen, and sweaty if sympathetic tone is increased, mottled blue and cold if sympathetic tone is decreased, or it may be normal. The skin often is hyperesthetic but, unlike the picture of true nerve damage, the hyperesthesia has a variable border. Unless the swelling is severe, or the problem long-standing, range of motion will be normal. These patients are very compliant when being examined and will use the affected limb even when they say they have not been able to use it recently. Conversion symptoms, such as numbness and paralysis, are unusual.

Additional Studies

Once the physician has seen a few of these adolescents and considers RND in the differential diagnosis, the diagnosis is not difficult to make on the basis of history, physical, and the dynamics of the physician-patient-parent interaction during examination. Diagnosis does not require sophisticated imaging techniques. In fact, images of the involved part are usually normal. Nevertheless, these patients often arrive in the sports medicine specialist's office carrying extensive paperwork

and images from previous workups that have revealed no diagnosis. Radiographs may reveal osteopenia if increased sympathetic tone has been long-standing. Technetium diphosphonate bone scans showing increased uptake of the involved part are said to be diagnostic of RND. However, increased uptake will be present only when the sympathetic tone is increased. When sympathetic tone is decreased, the scan may be normal or even show decreased uptake.[15] In Sherry and associates'[13] study, 27% of those with a psychosomatic problem had decreased uptake on bone scan.

Pain scales and psychologic interviews and tests of both the patient and family often reveal the underlying problems and the relative enmeshment.

Treatment

The treatment usually is not in the domain of the orthopaedic surgeon, and it may be difficult to find someone in the medical community who is familiar with this problem and who can proceed with testing as well as treatment. A multidisciplinary approach is required for best results. The principles of treatment include education, physical therapy, and counseling. The message that the original injury is over must be reinforced mentally as well as physically. The education process should include an explanation of the wiring of the nervous system and how the wires can become "short circuited" (Fig. 43). When the problem is described in this way, the patient does not carry the stigma of thinking the problem is "in her head." Supervised physical therapy is critical, because it is necessary to restore normal sympathetic tone, range of motion, and muscle strength in a patient who is unlikely to rehabilitate on her own. In addition, supervised therapy makes it obvious that the limb can, in fact, function.

When the problem is diagnosed early, normal sympathetic tone can be restored by purposefully stimulating the involved limb with temperature changes, sensory stimuli, and muscle use. Contrast therapy helps restore appropriate vasodilatation and vasoconstriction responses to temperature changes. Although sympathetic blocks, either via spinal anesthesia or oral medication, are sometimes necessary in adults with posttraumatic reflex sympathetic dystrophy, they are rarely necessary in the adolescent patient with RND or its psychosomatic variant. Sensory stimulation, such as massage, rubbing the skin with a

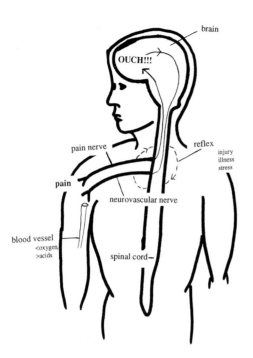

FIGURE 43
Reflex neurodystrophy schematic showing short circuiting of peripheral nerve input and response.

rough material such as a loofah sponge, or, for the foot, stepping barefooted in sand or small pebbles, ultimately decreases dysesthesia. Psychosocial counseling is usually required for both the patient and the family. Some patients are hospitalized for treatment. These in-patient programs include continuous individually supervised aerobic exercise for 5 hours daily, in addition to desensitization and appropriate psychotherapy. It is interesting that despite their complaints of pain, these patients are very compliant with a rigorous exercise program.

REFERENCES

1. Clapp JF III: A clinical approach to exercise during pregnancy. *Clin Sports Med* 1994;13:443-458.

2. American College of Obstetrics and Gynecology: Exercise during pregnancy and the postpartum period. Technical Bulletin No. 189, Feb 1994.

3. Holloway JB, Baechle TR: Strength training for female athletes: A review of selected aspects. *Sports Med* 1990;9:216-228.

4. Lopiano DA: Gender equity in sports, in Agostini R, Titus S (eds): *Medical and Orthopaedic Issues of Active and Athletic Women*. Philadelphia, PA, Hanley & Belfus, 1994, pp 13-22.

5. Baechle TR: Women in resistance training. *Clin Sports Med* 1984;3:791-808.

6. Corbin CB: Self-confidence of females in sports and physical activity. *Clin Sports Med* 1984;3:895-908.

7. Higginson DC: The influence of socializing agents in the female sport-participation process. *Adolescence* 1985;20:73-82.

8. Stuhr RM: Exercise prescription for women, in Agostini R, Titus S (eds): *Medical and Orthopaedic Issues of Active and Athletic Women*. Philadelphia, PA, Hanley & Belfus, 1994, pp 56-67.

9. Barnett NP, Wright P: Psychosocial factors and the developing female athlete, in Agostini R, Titus S (eds): *Medical and Orthopaedic Issues of Active and Athletic Women*. Philadelphia, PA, Hanley & Belfus, 1994, pp 92-101.

10. Sinclair DA, Orlick T: Positive transitions from high-performance sport. *Sport Psychologist* 1993;7:138-150.

11. Bernstein BH, Singsen BH, Kent JT, et al: Reflex neurovascular dystrophy in childhood. *J Pediatr* 1978;93:211-215.

12. Sherry DD, Weisman R: Psychologic aspects of childhood reflex neurovascular dystrophy. *Pediatrics* 1988;81:572-578.

13. Sherry DD, McGuire T, Mellins E, et al: Psychosomatic musculoskeletal pain in childhood: Clinical and psychological analyses of 100 children. *Pediatrics* 1991;88:1093-1099.

14. Smoll FL, Smith RE: Psychology of the young athlete: Stress-related maladies and remedial approaches. *Pediatr Clin North Am* 1990;37:1021-1046.

15. Laxer RM, Allen RC, Malleson PN, et al: Technetium 99m-methylene diphosphonate bone scans in children with reflex neurovascular dystrophy. *J Pediatr* 1985;106:437-440.

INDEX